S0-BZJ-273

Fundamentals of Cardiac Pacing

Anne B. Curtis, MD, FHRS, FACC, FAHA

Professor of Medicine
Chief, Division of Cardiology
Director of Cardiovascular Services
University of South Florida
Tampa, FL

JONES AND BARTLETT PUBLISHERS
Sudbury, Massachusetts
BOSTON   TORONTO   LONDON   SINGAPORE

World Headquarters
Jones and Bartlett Publishers
40 Tall Pine Drive
Sudbury, MA 01776
978-443-5000
info@jbpub.com
www.jbpub.com

Jones and Bartlett Publishers
Canada
6339 Ormindale Way
Mississauga, Ontario L5V 1J2
Canada

Jones and Bartlett Publishers
International
Barb House, Barb Mews
London W6 7PA
United Kingdom

Jones and Bartlett's books and products are available through most bookstores and online booksellers. To contact Jones and Bartlett Publishers directly, call 800-832-0034, fax 978-443-8000, or visit our website www.jbpub.com.

Substantial discounts on bulk quantities of Jones and Bartlett's publications are available to corporations, professional associations, and other qualified organizations. For details and specific discount information, contact the special sales department at Jones and Bartlett via the above contact information or send an email to specialsales@jbpub.com.

Copyright © 2010 by Jones and Bartlett Publishers, LLC

All rights reserved. No part of the material protected by this copyright may be reproduced or utilized in any form, electronic or mechanical, including photocopying, recording, or by any information storage and retrieval system, without written permission from the copyright owner.

The authors, editor, and publisher have made every effort to provide accurate information. However, they are not responsible for errors, omissions, or for any outcomes related to the use of the contents of this book and take no responsibility for the use of the products and procedures described. Treatments and side effects described in this book may not be applicable to all people; likewise, some people may require a dose or experience a side effect that is not described herein. Drugs and medical devices are discussed that may have limited availability controlled by the Food and Drug Administration (FDA) for use only in a research study or clinical trial. Research, clinical practice, and government regulations often change the accepted standard in this field. When consideration is being given to use of any drug in the clinical setting, the healthcare provider or reader is responsible for determining FDA status of the drug, reading the package insert, and reviewing prescribing information for the most up-to-date recommendations on dose, precautions, and contraindications, and determining the appropriate usage for the product. This is especially important in the case of drugs that are new or seldom used.

Production Credits
Senior Acquisitions Editor: Alison Hankey
Senior Editorial Assistant: Jessica Acox
Production Director: Amy Rose
Production Assistant: Laura Almozara
Marketing Manager: Ilana Goddess
V.P., Manufacturing and Inventory Control: Therese Connell
Composition: Paw Print Media
Cover Design: Kristin E. Parker
Cover Images: Top image: © Rasch, Shuttershock, Inc.; Bottom image: © Bocosb, Dreamstime.com
Cover Printing: Malloy, Inc.
Printing and Binding: Malloy, Inc.

Library of Congress Cataloging-in-Publication Data
Curtis, Anne B.
 Fundamentals of cardiac pacing / Anne B. Curtis.
   p. ; cm.
 Includes bibliographical references and index.
 ISBN-13: 978-0-7637-5630-7
 ISBN-10: 0-7637-5630-X
 1. Cardiac pacing. I. Title.
 [DNLM: 1. Cardiac Pacing, Artificial—methods. 2. Pacemaker, Artificial. WG 168 C9785 2010]
 RC684.P3C873 2010
 617.4'120645—dc22
                          2008048276

6048

Printed in the United States of America
13 12 11 10 09   10 9 8 7 6 5 4 3 2 1

To my husband, Alexander Domijan, Jr., PhD.
Thank you for all your love and support.

Contents

Acronym Key

ADL	Activities of Daily Living
AF	Atrial Fibrillation
AMS	Automatic Mode Switching
ATP	Antitachycardia Pacing
AV	Atrioventricular
BOL	Beginning of Life
BOS	Beginning of Service
$CHADS_2$	Congestive Heart Failure/Hypertension/Age > 75 years/Diabetes Mellitus/Previous Stroke or Transient Ischemic Attack
CRT	Cardiac Resynchronization Therapy
CS	Coronary Sinus
DBS	Drawn Brazen Strand
DFT	Drawn Filled Tube
ECG	Electrocardiogram
EGM	Electrogram
ELT	Endless Loop Tachycardia
EMI	Electromagnetic Interference
EOL	End of Life
EOS	End of Service
ERI	Elective Replacement Indicator
IBM	Internet-Based Monitoring
IC	Integrated Circuit
ICD	Implantable Cardioverter Defibrillator
IVC	Inferior Vena Cava
LAO	Left Anterior Oblique; Fluoroscopy View
LBBB	Left Bundle Branch Block
LRL	Lower Rate Limit
LVEF	Left Ventricular Ejection Fraction
NYHA	New York Heart Association

OTW	Over-The-Wire (Leads)
PAC	Premature Atrial Contraction
PMT	Pacemaker-Mediated Tachycardia
PVARP	Post Ventricular Atrial Refractory Period
PVC	Premature Ventricular Contraction
RAA	Right Atrial Appendage
RAO	Right Anterior Oblique; Fluoroscopy View
RBBB	Right Bundle Branch Block
RRT	Recommended Replacement Time
RVA	Right Ventricular Apex
SA	Sinoatrial
SPWMD	Septal-to-Posterior-Wall Motion Delay
SVC	Superior Vena Cava
TARP	Total Atrial Refractory Period
TTM	Transtelephonic Pacemaker Monitoring
URL	Upper Rate Limit
VT	Ventricular Tachycardia

Preface

Having been involved in the teaching of cardiac electrophysiology and pacing for over twenty years, it is a pleasure to be able to put the key concepts in cardiac pacing into one concise textbook.

This book is intended as an introduction to the subject of cardiac pacing for those who have little to no background in the field. It would be suitable for physicians, cardiology fellows, residents, and other fellows who want to know more about pacemakers, as well as nurses, other allied professionals, electrophysiology laboratory personnel, and students in medicine and other medical fields. No background knowledge in this area is assumed, yet by the time one is finished reading the book, one should be well grounded in the indications for pacemakers, details of implantation techniques, technology of pacemaker leads and generators, basic and advanced programming, and troubleshooting and follow-up. There are also basic chapters on the cardiac conduction system, rate-responsive pacing, cardiac resynchronization therapy, and complications of pacemaker implantation. There is an introductory chapter on the history of pacing that will provide an indication of the remarkable progress we have seen in the field of cardiac pacing over a relatively short period of time.

I would like to thank my co-authors, Dr. Gustavo Lopera and Dr. Robert Hariman, for their excellent contributions to the book. I would especially like to thank Dr. Lopera for contributing a number of figures in other chapters from his own clinical practice.

My hope is that upon finishing the book, the reader will feel comfortable with the basic management of patients who need or have cardiac pacemakers, and perhaps that his or her interest will be stimulated enough to want to pursue further knowledge in this fascinating field.

Anne B. Curtis

List of Contributors

Robert J. Hariman, MD, FACC
Professor of Medicine
University of South Florida
Chief, Cardiology Section
James A. Haley VA Medical Center
Tampa, Florida

Gustavo Lopera, MD, FHRS, FACC
Assistant Professor of Clinical Medicine
University of Miami/Miller School of Medicine
Director, Arrhythmia Service
Miami Veterans Affairs Health Care System

1 ▪ A Brief History of Cardiac Pacing

Permanent pacing is now so routine that it is almost difficult to imagine a time when patients with complete atrioventricular (AV) block would suffer repeated syncopal spells (Stokes-Adams attacks) and even death, because there was no treatment available for severe bradycardia or asystole. The development of permanent pacing required visionary thinking by a number of physicians and engineers, often in the face of substantial skepticism as to the feasibility and safety of a permanently implantable cardiac pacing system.

Electrocardiography and the Physiology of Heart Block

The clinical presentation of patients with heart block was described by Drs. William Stokes and Robert Adams in the mid-nineteenth century. They recognized the slow pulse and the disconnection between the peripheral pulses and the rate at which the heart beats when listening with a stethoscope. However, at the time, electrocardiography had not yet been invented, and so their insights were limited to the physical examination and findings at autopsy, which were few.

By the late nineteenth century, it was understood that electrical activity was involved in the heart beating. The British physiologist Augustus Waller recorded electrical variations in the heartbeat, but he did not understand the meaning of the signals, and his capillary electrometer was too complex to use outside of a laboratory setting. Another physiologist, Walter Gaskell, demonstrated that myocardial contraction occurred due to a wave of electrical impulses that traversed the heart, and that creation of a slit between the atria and the ventricles would make it more difficult for the contraction wave to pass to the ventricles. Subsequently, Willem Einthoven, a physiologist at the University of Leiden, developed modern electrocardiography by building on the work of Waller. He developed the string galvanometer, the forerunner of modern electrocardiographic (ECG) equipment, and he was able to relate physiologic events to observations on the ECG. Stokes-Adams attacks were then recognized to be due to failure of impulses in the atria to reach the ventricles, a condition demonstrated on the ECG that came to be known as complete AV block, or heart block. The recognition that failure of impulse propagation in the heart could lead to the severe symptoms and even death associated with Stokes-Adams attacks naturally led to interest in correcting the problem by artificially providing electrical stimulation to the heart.

The development of electrocardiography by Dr. Willem Einthoven led to a better understanding of the physiology of Stokes-Adams attacks by correlation of physical findings with observations on the ECG.

Electrical Stimulation of the Heart

The earliest demonstration of temporary pacing of the heart was provided by Mark C. Lidwill in the 1920s. Dr. Lidwill developed a portable piece of electrical equipment that was meant to provide temporary pacing in the event of an emergency during a surgical procedure. The equipment plugged into a standard wall socket and delivered electrical pulses to the heart by means of a pad placed on the skin that was saturated with salt solution, and a needle plunged directly into the heart. He used it successfully to revive a stillborn infant in Australia.

Albert S. Hyman was the next major figure in the development of cardiac pacing. Dr. Hyman obtained a patent in 1930 for a device with a spring motor and a hand crank that employed a needle electrode that would be plunged directly into the heart between the ribs. Technical problems rendered the device unsuccessful in most applications. In addition, the medical community considered asystole to be a rare and hopeless situation for which cardiac pacing was highly unlikely to be useful.

There was little further progress in the development of pacing until the 1950s. At that time, a research group from the Banting Institute in Toronto, Canada (John Callaghan, Wilfred Bigelow, and Jack Hopps) developed an external pulse generator and an electrode that could be introduced into the heart via the right internal jugular vein. They attempted to use it in a few hospitalized patients in 1950, but they failed, most likely because they placed the electrode in the atrium rather than the ventricle, which would be ineffective in complete AV block. Dr. Paul Zoll learned of the external pacemaker and worked on his own version by using a standard physiologic stimulator. He successfully used his stimulator with external needle electrodes on a patient in 1952 who presented with AV block.

Shortly thereafter, in 1954, Electrodyne came out with a commercial version of an external pacemaker. These devices came into widespread use in hospitals throughout the 1950s for the emergency resuscitation of patients with asystole.

With the development of open heart surgery around this same time, postsurgical heart block became a vexing problem; for example, after repair of congenital abnormalities such as ventricular septal defects. Two trainees of Dr. C. Walton Lillehei, Drs. Vincent Gott and William Weirich, employing the same type of physiologic stimulator used by Zoll, developed a technique for epicardial pacing using a wire sewn onto the ventricle. It was first used successfully on a young girl in 1957. A battery-powered external pacemaker generator was subsequently developed by Earl Bakken, the founder of Medtronic, Inc., using transistors, small batteries, and a circuit design for a metronome he had seen in an electronics magazine.

While these results were gratifying, external pacemakers were only practical for temporary use. It quickly became apparent that chronic pacing would best be achieved with a totally implantable system.

> The first attempts at cardiac pacing involved external generators that were intended to resuscitate patients in emergencies or after heart surgery. The earliest electrodes were plunge electrodes meant to be introduced to the heart directly, or external patch electrodes.

Permanent Pacemaker Implantation

An engineer named Norman Roth developed a permanent epicardial pacing lead in the late 1950s. It was first implanted on April 14, 1959, by Dr. Samuel Hunter in St. Paul, Minnesota, in a patient named Warren Mauston. The lead was attached to the same model 5800 Medtronic pacemaker generator that was being used at the time for temporary applications. Mr. Mauston survived for over 6 years with his external pacemaker generator. The original lead lasted for 4 years before it was replaced with a transvenous lead.

Around this time, several groups were working on a totally implantable pacing system. There were multiple technical challenges to overcome: a totally implantable system to avoid infection; a generator small enough to implant in the body; a battery that would last a reasonable length of time or be rechargeable; a lead that would not break easily with the repeated flexing caused by the beating heart and also have a stable pacing threshold; and appropriate circuitry that could be shielded from body fluids.

In addition to the names just mentioned, two other groups involved in the first implantable pacing systems should be recognized. The first permanent pacemaker was implanted by Dr. Ake Senning in Sweden in 1958 in a patient named Arne Larsson. It was a totally implantable system that used an epicardial lead on the ventricle. The pacemaker was developed by an engineer named Rune Elmqvist, using electrical parameters that had been determined from observations of external pacing in patients with complete AV block. The system used large nickel-cadmium cells to power the pacemaker, and it lasted only a matter of hours before it needed to be replaced. Subsequent pacemakers lasted months before replacements were needed. The batteries were rechargeable and used a radiofrequency induction coil for recharging. Mr. Larsson actually had 26 pacemakers throughout his life, starting with the original Ni-Cd battery, through mercury-zinc technology, and ending with his last generator in 1993 that was a lithium-iodine battery. The story of Arne Larsson provides an excellent testimonial to the success of permanent pacing. After having suffered from multiple daily syncopal spells just before he received his first pacemaker, the patient went on to lead a full and productive life, until he died in 2001 at the age of 86.

The first permanent pacemaker implantation in the United States was performed in Buffalo, New York, in a patient named Frank Henefelt by Dr. William Chardack in 1960, using an epicardial lead and a pacemaker generator constructed by Wilson Greatbatch. After having suffered repeated Stokes-Adams attacks before the implantation, Mr. Henefelt recovered uneventfully and lived for 30 months with the implanted pacemaker. Major milestones in the development of permanent pacing are shown in **Figure 1.1**.

> **Arne Larsson received the first totally implantable permanent pacemaker in Sweden in 1958. The nickel-cadmium batteries required monthly recharging, and generator changes were required much more often than is the case today.**

Transvenous Pacing

Pacemaker electrodes were initially placed by thoracotomy. Dr. Seymour Furman, one of the giants of cardiac pacing and a founder of the North American Society of Pacing and Electrophysiology

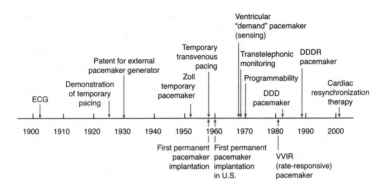

■ Figure 1.1   Major milestones in cardiac pacing

(now known as the Heart Rhythm Society), developed the first practical temporary transvenous pacing lead. He first implanted it in a human in 1958; the generator to which it was attached was large enough to require a cart when the patient walked around. Dr. Furman was responsible for other advances in the field of cardiac pacing. He pioneered the use of the cephalic vein cut-down technique for lead implantation. In addition, the concept of transtelephonic monitoring of pacemakers was developed by Dr. Furman around 1968. Given the short battery life of pacemakers in the 1960s, remote monitoring was important for safety reasons to pick up impending battery depletion.

The first totally implantable, transvenous, permanent pacemaker system was implanted in 1962 by surgeon Hans Lagergren from the Karolinska Hospital in Stockholm, Sweden.

> **The first practical temporary transvenous pacing lead was developed by Dr. Seymour Furman, one of the founders of the North American Society of Pacing and Electrophysiology (now known as the Heart Rhythm Society).**

Power Sources

The original power source in permanent pacemaker generators was the mercury-zinc battery, but there were several problems inherent with this technology. First, the batteries produced hydrogen gas that had to be dissipated, preventing hermetic sealing of the generator. These batteries also wore out quickly, often in 18 months or less. Most importantly, they could fail unexpectedly because of short circuits or damage to the circuitry from sodium hydroxide produced in the chemical reaction. Dr. Victor Parsonnet, another one of the founders of what is now the Heart Rhythm Society, studied alternative energy sources for pacemakers. He implanted the first nuclear pacemaker in the United States in 1973. Nuclear pacemakers were implanted for a few years in the 1970s, but they were quickly supplanted by lithium iodine batteries, which have been the standard in pacemaker generators ever since (**Figure 1.2**).

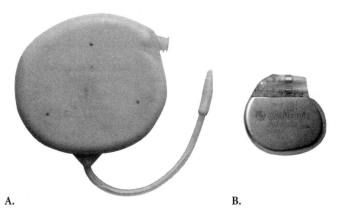

A.   B.

■ **Figure 1.2   Pacemaker generators**

A. A Chardack-Greatbatch generator from 1960.

B. A dual-chamber pacemaker generator from 2008, showing the remarkable reduction in size while the technology has become much more sophisticated.

Courtesy of Medtronic, Inc.

Technological Developments

The first pacemakers were very simple systems that paced the ventricle asynchronously at a fixed rate, initially 72 beats per minute. They could sustain life in patients with complete AV block, but were very limited in other regards. Sensing was not possible, nor was atrial pacing, or other features healthcare providers now take for granted. In fact, the fixed rate and lack of sensing could lead to ventricular fibrillation in some cases, because pacing stimuli fell in the vulnerable period of the patient's own heartbeat. Until the problem of reliable sensing of cardiac activity was solved, pacemakers could only be implanted in patients who were 100 percent dependent on pacing. The first ventricular demand pacemaker, invented by Barouh Berkovits, was implanted in 1966 in a patient with intermittent heart block. Around the same time, Wilson Greatbatch also developed a demand pacemaker that was implanted by Dr. Chardack in 1966 or late 1965. Demand pacing indicates that pacing impulses are delivered only when there is a need, or "demand," for pacing because of bradycardia or asystole, with sensed signals inhibiting pacing the remainder of the time.

The first AV synchronous pacemaker, which stimulated the ventricle off a sensed P wave, was developed by the Cordis Corporation by Walt Keller and implanted in a patient in 1962 by Dr. Sol Center in New York. Several companies then rushed to develop fully functional dual-chamber pacemakers. The first dual-chamber pacemakers that achieved atrial pacing actually worked in the DVI mode (see Chapter 5); that is, they paced the atrium and the ventricle but were inhibited if there was spontaneous ventricular activity. Subsequently, Cordis introduced the Sequicor pacemaker, a DDD pacemaker that could sense and pace both chambers, in 1982.

The development of totally transvenous dual-chamber pacemakers required that leads be developed that could be implanted transvenously in the atrium, specifically a "J" shape for stability in the right atrial appendage (RAA). In addition, the pacemaker circuitry had to be capable of sensing the smaller signals found in the atrium. The algorithms for pacing and sensing, as well as the timing, become much more complex in a dual-chamber system compared to a single-chamber pacemaker.

Asynchronous, fixed-rate ventricular pacemakers were quickly supplanted by "demand" pacemakers that could sense ventricular activity and inhibit pacing. Dual-chamber pacemakers followed later, with atrial sensing and pacing requiring further technical developments.

Rate-responsive pacemakers were developed in the 1980s. Until that time, a change in heart rate above the base pacing rate was only possible with atrial tracking. With permanent atrial fibrillation (AF), tracking of atrial activation is not desirable because it may lead to rapid, irregular ventricular rates. With sinus bradycardia, even if atrial activation is tracked reliably, the ventricular rate cannot increase beyond the sinus rate and exercise tolerance may thus be compromised. The invention of sensors that used activity or some physiologic parameter to detect exertion on the part of the patient led to the development of rate-responsive pacemakers. Single-chamber rate-responsive pacemakers that used body motion as the sensor were first available in 1981; dual-chamber rate-responsive pacemakers came along in 1989.

Developments in lead technology have been just as important to the widespread use of pacemakers as advances in battery design and circuitry. The overwhelming majority of pacemakers are implanted transvenously. In the early days, high dislodgement rates and high pacing thresholds were significant problems. An important early development was the coiled spring lead designed by Dr. William Chardack. New designs for electrode fixation, both passive and active fixation, have helped to minimize dislodgement rates. Improvements in electrode design have also helped to reduce acute and chronic pacing thresholds. A major advance in reducing pacing thresholds has been the development of steroid-eluting leads (see Chapter 4).

More recently, cardiac resynchronization therapy (CRT) for the management of heart failure has become widespread (see Chapter 13). CRT required the development of leads for pacing the left ventricle via the coronary sinus (CS). The major design challenge with these leads was the requirement for a stable position without the use of existing fixation methods such as tines or screws that would not be advisable for long-term use in a venous system. In addition, more complex pacing algorithms and triple-chamber generators had to be developed.

Although there has also been investigation into triple-site pacing in which biatrial or dual-site atrial pacing is used for the prevention of atrial tachyarrhythmias, this approach has not proven to be nearly as successful as CRT and has largely been abandoned.

Major milestones in permanent pacing include the first pacemaker implantations in the 1950s, multiprogrammability in the 1960s, dual-chamber pacing in the 1970s, rate-responsive pacing in the 1980s, and CRT in the early twenty-first century.

Programmability

The initial fixed-rate, asynchronous ventricular pacemakers were nonprogrammable. The first advance in programmability was the ability to change rate and output voltage, although it had to be done invasively. The development of more complex functions in permanent pacemakers required the ability to change pacing parameters after implantation. Such programming was made feasible in the 1970s because of two developments: integrated circuits (IC) and the advent of radiofrequency communication between the implanted pacemaker generator and an external programmer.

Conclusion

The rapid technological development of permanent pacemakers over the past 50 years has allowed millions of patients to benefit from these devices. They have proven to be both lifesaving as well as instrumental in improving quality of life in many patients with bradyarrhythmias. What the medical field now takes for granted as a routine part of modern cardiac patient care is the result of the foresight and creativity of the important pioneers in cardiac pacing.

Suggested Readings

Greatbatch W. *The Making of the Pacemaker*. Amherst, NY: Prometheus Books; 2000.

Jeffrey K. *Machines in Our Hearts: The Cardiac Pacemaker, The Implantable Defibrillator, and American Health Care*. Baltimore, MD: Johns Hopkins University Press; 2001.

Luderitz B. Historical perspectives on interventional electrophysiology. *J Interv Cardiac Electrophysiol*. 2003;9:75–83.

2 ■ The Cardiac Conduction System

The Cardiac Action Potential

All cardiac cells have a semipermeable membrane that allows the flow of ions into and out of the cells. Sodium (Na^+), potassium (K^+), and calcium (Ca^{2+}) are the most important ions involved in the cardiac action potential, with smaller contributions by other ions. Proteins embedded in the cell membranes form channels that allow ions to flow into and out of the cells. These channels have gating mechanisms that may be open, closed, or inactivated, depending on the membrane potential at any point in time. There are also ion pumps that actively work to move ions into or out of the cells to control the membrane potential. In normal cardiac cells, there is a much higher concentration of K^+ inside the cells and a much higher concentration of Na^+ ions outside the cells. This natural imbalance creates an electrical potential across the cell, which can be measured in millivolts (mV). Normal myocardium has a resting potential around -90 mV.

> The difference in K^+ concentrations inside and outside cardiac cells and the greater permeability of the cell membrane under quiescent conditions to K^+ are responsible for the normal resting potential of -90 mV.

When an electrical impulse reaches a cell in the specialized conduction system or the myocardium, Na channels start to open, allowing Na^+ to start flowing into the cell. This flow of ions causes depolarization of the cell until it reaches the threshold potential (approximately -60 mV). At this point, Na channels open rapidly, causing a massive influx of Na^+ ions into the cell. This rapid inward current is responsible for phase 0 of the cardiac action potential (**Figure 2.1**). Phase 0 is followed by phase 1, the early rapid repolarization phase, which is controlled predominantly by

13

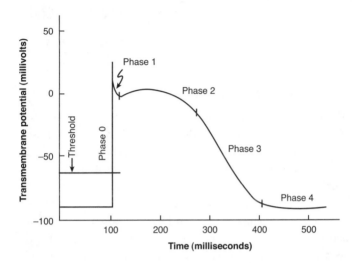

■ Figure 2.1   Cardiac action potential from a Purkinje fiber

Phase 0 is the rapid depolarization phase, due to rapid influx of Na^+ ions into the cell. This is followed by phase 1, early rapid repolarization; phase 2, the plateau phase; and phase 3, repolarization. Phase 4 is the slow, spontaneous depolarization phase. Action potentials in the atria and the ventricles are similar in shape, with differences in the rate of phase 0 depolarization and the duration of the action potential.

a transient outward K^+ current (I_{to}), an outward chloride (Cl^-) current, as well as inactivation of the inward Na^+ current. Phase 2 is the plateau phase of the cardiac action potential, and it is controlled in part by a slow inward Ca^{2+} current. There are also other currents that contribute to the plateau current, including a slowly activating Na^+ current, several K^+ currents, a Cl^- current, and ion-exchange pumps.

The repolarization phase of the action potential, phase 3, is controlled primarily by several K^+ currents, which have different properties and different kinetics. Once the cell returns to its resting potential, there is a slow, spontaneous depolarization called phase 4 that occurs even in the absence of electrical excitation from neighboring cells. This spontaneous depolarization is most characteristic of sinoatrial (SA) and AV nodal cells. In the SA node, there is a hyperpolarization-activated current called I_f (for "funny") that is responsible for phase 4 depolarization. The slow depolarization in phase 4 will eventually allow the cell to reach the threshold potential, starting the process of depolarization and repolarization all over again. This process of spontaneous depolarization is the basis for automaticity in the heart, leading to automatic impulse initiation. The rate at which these depolarizations occur depends on the slope of phase 4. The slope of phase 4 may be altered in various ways; for example, circulating catecholamines will lead to a steeper slope of phase 4 and thus a more rapid heartbeat.

A wide variety of drugs affect repolarization, mostly by virtue of their effects on K^+ currents. Repolarization is reflected on the ECG by the QT interval. When drugs or electrolyte imbalances prolong the QT interval, ventricular arrhythmias such as torsades de pointes may result.

The shape of the action potential for SA and AV nodal cells is quite different from that of other cardiac cells (**Figure 2.2**). One reason for the difference is the fact that the slow inward Ca^{2+} current is predominately responsible for depolarization in these cells, leading to a much slower phase 0 than is found in other cardiac cells. The difference in the slope of phase 4 depolarization is also striking. In addition, the resting membrane potential in SA and AV nodal cells is more depolarized (around -60 mV) compared to the rest of the heart. These differences between SA and AV nodal cells and the rest of the heart's specialized conduction system and myocardium explain some of the variation in the effects of cardiac drugs in different regions of the heart. For example, beta blockers directly affect phase 4 depolarization, and thus they have their most pronounced effects on the SA node, where the spontaneous rate of phase 4 depolarization is greatest. Also, Ca channel blockers have a greater effect on the SA and AV nodes than in the rest of

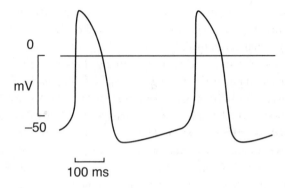

■ Figure 2.2 Cardiac action potential from the SA or AV node

Note that the resting potential is less negative than in the Purkinje fiber. Phase 0 is less rapid, while phase 4 depolarization is faster.

the heart because of the importance of the slow inward Ca^{2+} current in these cells.

> The SA and AV nodes have a less-negative resting membrane potential, higher rate of spontaneous depolarization, and slower upstroke of depolarization compared to other cells in the heart.

ECG Correlates of the Action Potential

The signals recorded from the surface ECG correspond to the progression of action potentials in the heart. The P wave correlates with atrial depolarization and repolarization. The PR interval reflects conduction time through the atria and the AV node. The QRS complex correlates with ventricular depolarization, while the T wave corresponds to ventricular repolarization. Delays in conduction through the His-Purkinje system are manifested as intraventricular conduction delays or bundle branch block.

Automaticity and Impulse Propagation

The SA node is the heart's natural pacemaker, since it has the steepest slope for phase 4, and thus the most rapid firing. Other cells can fire spontaneously as well, but the slope of phase 4 is shallower, leading to slower firing. However, if the SA node ceases to fire, permanently or temporarily, these subsidiary pacemakers can take over. For example, the AV node tends to fire at rates around 50 beats per minute. It will be suppressed under conditions of normal SA node function, but it may become evident under conditions of sinus arrest. The more distal in the conduction system one goes, the slower the spontaneous depolarization of the cells, so that ventricular myocardium may only fire at rates around 30 beats per minute. All of these behaviors are considered normal automaticity in the heart. Abnormal automaticity may occur under conditions of ischemia, for example, or for unclear reasons in various pathological tachycardias (rapid heartbeats). In these cases, even though the SA node is capable of firing normally, these abnormal, rapid depolarizations in other parts of the heart control the heartbeat and lead to suppression of SA node function.

> The cardiac cells with the most rapid phase 4 depolarization will have the fastest rate of firing and serve as the heart's pacemaker. Under normal circumstances, the SA node fulfills this role.

Normal impulses that arise in the SA node must be conducted through the rest of the heart. Cells in the heart are arranged longitudinally so that conduction can occur in a rapid fashion from the SA node down through to the ventricles. At the end of each cell, there are intercalated discs, known as gap junctions, that allow the electrical signals to jump quickly to the next cell in sequence. The orientation of myocardial fibers and the function of the gap junctions promote longitudinal conduction to a much greater degree than side-to-side conduction. The result of this process under normal circumstances is rapid impulse propagation throughout the heart with minimal chance for lateral conduction of electrical impulses and subsequent promotion of reentrant tachyarrhythmias.

Anisotropy is the term used to refer to the fact that conduction in the heart is much more rapid in a longitudinal direction parallel to the orientation of muscle fibers than transversely.

Anatomy of the Conduction System

Comprised of two upper chambers (atria) and two lower chambers (ventricles), the heart pumps blood through the body by an organized sequence of contraction of the atria followed by the ventricles. In order for the muscle cells of the heart, the myocytes, to contract, they must be activated by electrical signals, a process called electromechanical coupling. The flow of electrical signals through the heart causes depolarization of the myocytes, leading to contraction of the individual cells. However, the velocity of conduction of electrical signals through the myocytes is relatively slow. If this were the only means by which electricity is conducted through the heart, cells in the upper regions of each chamber would contract well before impulses reach the lower regions. The result would be an uncoordinated and inefficient contraction of the cardiac chambers, compromising cardiac output.

In order to create synchronized contraction of the heart, there is a specialized conduction system in the heart that conducts electrical impulses rapidly, allowing myocytes throughout the heart to be depolarized nearly simultaneously for the most efficient pumping action. The conduction system consists of the SA node, specialized conduction pathways through the atria, the AV node, and the His-Purkinje system (see **Figure 2.3**).

The specialized conduction system is responsible for rapid conduction of electrical impulses throughout the atria and the ventricles.

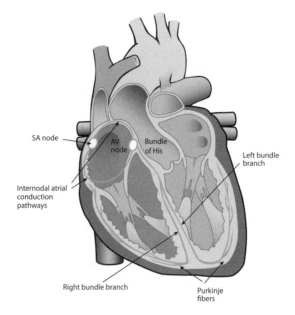

■ **Figure 2.3 Specialized conduction system**

Spontaneous impulses arise in the SA node, travel through the atria, converging on the AV node. From there, the electrical impulses conduct through the His-Purkinje system and rapidly depolarize the ventricles.

The SA node is a collection of specialized cells in the upper part of the right atrium. Spontaneous depolarization here leads to electrical signals conducting through the atria. While all cells in the atria will depolarize, there are preferential pathways by which impulses are conducted more rapidly. For example, Bachmann's bundle, located in the anteroseptal portion of the interatrial septum, allows rapid conduction of electrical impulses to the left atrium.

Impulses from the atria will eventually reach the AV node, which is normally the only electrical connection between the atria and the ventricles. While conduction throughout the atria is rapid in the normal heart, allowing near-simultaneous depolarization of both atria for the most coordinated contraction, conduction through the AV node is relatively slow. It usually takes 80 milliseconds (msec) or more for impulses to travel through the AV node. This slowing down or natural braking action in the AV node has a couple of important benefits. Not only does it allow time for the atria to complete contraction before the ventricles are activated, but the slow conduction serves as a filter for impulses from the atria during tachyarrhythmias. For example, AF, a rapid, disorganized atrial arrhythmia, may reach rates well over 300 beats per minute. The AV node will typically not allow more than half those impulses to reach the ventricles, leading to ventricular rates during AF that are no more than 150 beats per minute in most cases. This filtering action is cardio-protective, because much more rapid rates could lead to collapse and even death.

The AV node conducts impulses relatively slowly, allowing atrial contraction to be completed before depolarization of the ventricles commences.

As electrical impulses exit the AV node, they travel through the His bundle and then through the Purkinje system. The His bundle is a relatively thick bundle in the anteroseptal region at the junction between the atria and the ventricles. It quickly branches into a left bundle branch and a right bundle branch. The left bundle branch subdivides into an anterior and a posterior branch. These bundle branches then subdivide further and further into small fibers that branch out throughout the endocardium. Conduction in the His-Purkinje system is quite rapid (3–4 m/sec). By having this specialized conduction system in the ventricles, electrical impulses are quickly conducted to every region of the ventricles. Although muscle-to-muscle conduction of electrical impulses is also possible, the process is so slow (on the order of 0.3–1 m/sec) that coordinated contraction of the ventricles would not be possible without the presence of this specialized conduction system.

Conduction System Disorders

Conduction disorders that lead to a need for permanent pacing are due to a failure of impulse initiation or propagation, or both. In the SA node, progressive fibrosis, among other conditions, can lead to failure of impulse initiation (sinus arrest), failure of impulses to conduct out of the SA node to the atrium (sinus exit block), or slowing of spontaneous depolarization (sinus bradycardia). Patients who have sinus node dysfunction may also have failure to reach adequate heart rates with exercise, a condition known as chronotropic incompetence. In addition, many patients with sinus node dysfunction have the tendency to develop atrial arrhythmias such as atrial tachycardia, atrial flutter, and AF. The rapid rates associated with these arrhythmias lead to overdrive suppression of the SA node, so that when the tachyarrhythmias terminate, there is often a prolonged pause because of failure of the SA node to fire.

> Conduction disorders in the heart are primarily due to failure of adequate impulse initiation (e.g., sinus node dysfunction) or failure of impulse propagation through the heart (e.g., AV block).

The other major category of conduction system disorders is AV block. Impulses may be normally generated by the SA node and propagated through the atria, but blocks at various levels below that may prevent the impulses from reaching and depolarizing the ventricles. The various types and levels of AV block are discussed in greater detail in Chapter 3. Fundamentally, though, impulses may be slowed in their transmission to the ventricles (first-degree AV block), there may be intermittent block of some of the impulses from the atria to the ventricles (second-degree AV block, 2:1 AV block, and high-grade AV block), or all of the impulses from the atria may be blocked from transmission to the ventricles (third-degree or complete AV block).

Suggested Readings

Dobrzynski H, Boyett MR, Anderson RH. New insights into pacemaker activity: Promoting understanding of sick sinus syndrome. *Circulation.* 2007;115:1921–1932.

Rubart M, Zipes DP. Genesis of cardiac arrhythmias: Electrophysiological considerations. In: Libby P, Bonow RO, Mann DL, Zipes DP, eds. *Braunwald's Heart Disease: A Textbook of Cardiovascular Medicine*, 8th ed. Philadelphia: Elsevier Saunders; 2008:727–762.

Task Force of the Working Group on Arrhythmias of the European Society of Cardiology. The Sicilian gambit. A new approach to the classification of antiarrhythmic drugs based on their actions on arrhythmogenic mechanisms. *Circulation.* 1991;84:1831–1851.

3 ▪ Indications for Pacing

Indications for cardiac pacemakers have evolved dramatically from the early years of device therapy, when their size, rudimentary capabilities, and short battery life dictated that they be used exclusively in patients with AV block. Technology has advanced remarkably, with the development of smaller devices, multiprogrammability, and longer battery lives. In addition, clinical trials have demonstrated the value of permanent pacing in a variety of conditions beyond simple bradyarrhythmias. This information has been distilled into clinical guidelines documents that provide the best current recommendations for the implantation of permanent pacemakers.

ACC/AHA/HRS Guidelines

It is important to be familiar with published guidelines for pacemaker implantation. The most recent version is the *ACC/AHA/HRS 2008 Guidelines for Device-Based Therapy of Cardiac Rhythm Abnormalities*. In this document, as in all guidelines documents, class I indications are those conditions for which there is evidence and/or general agreement that a given procedure/therapy is beneficial, useful, and effective. Class II indications are those conditions for which there is conflicting evidence and/or a divergence of opinion about the usefulness/efficacy of performing the procedure/therapy. Class II indications are further subdivided into class IIa, for which the weight of evidence/opinion is in favor of usefulness/efficacy, and class IIb, in which usefulness/efficacy is less well established by evidence/opinion. Finally, class III represents conditions for which there is evidence and/or general agreement that a procedure/therapy is not useful or effective and in some cases may be harmful. Pacemakers are implanted in most cases for class I and IIa indications. Implantation for class IIb indications in some cases may be reasonable, particularly as practice advances in the light of new information from clinical trials.

However, pacemakers should not be implanted for class III indications.

> **Professional society guidelines give useful information as to currently accepted indications for permanent pacing. However, indications continue to evolve as new information is gleaned from clinical trials.**

It should be noted that, for the great majority of indications for pacemakers, symptoms are key. For example, an athlete may have a resting heart rate of 45 beats per minute because of excellent conditioning and have superb exercise tolerance and no symptoms. Clearly, a permanent pacemaker would not be indicated in such a situation. On the other hand, an elderly patient might have an inability to increase the heart rate to more than 70 beats per minute with exertion, an abnormal situation that would likely be associated with exercise intolerance. Such a condition, known as chronotropic incompetence, is a class I indication for permanent pacing. Symptoms that may be associated with indications for pacing include dizziness, syncope, dyspnea on exertion, fatigue, and exercise intolerance.

> **Symptoms govern whether cardiac pacing is indicated in most patients. Correlation of symptoms with bradyarrhythmias is thus important in deciding whether pacing is likely to be helpful in improving a patient's symptoms.**

Sinus Node Dysfunction

The most common indication for implantation of pacemakers in the United States is sinus node dysfunction. Also known as sick sinus syndrome, it is actually a disorder of the sinus node and the atria. Manifestations include sinus bradycardia (heart rate slower than 60 beats per minute), pauses in electrical impulse initiation that may be detected on an ECG as sinus arrest or SA exit block, chronotropic incompetence, and atrial tachyarrhythmias such as atrial tachycardia, atrial flutter, and AF. When sick sinus syndrome is associated with both bradycardia and tachycardia, it is called tachy-brady syndrome. Common definitions of chronotropic incompetence include a maximum heart rate less than 100 beats per minute, or failure to reach 70 percent of the maximum predicted heart rate (220 minus age in years) with exercise. Tachycardia and bradycardia are often both present in patients with sinus node dysfunction. Medications to manage the tachycardia may then aggravate any existing bradycardia, leading to the need for pacemaker implantation to control symptoms. Class I and IIa indications for permanent pacing in sinus node dysfunction are shown in **Table 3.1**.

The diagnosis of sinus node dysfunction is made by correlation of bradycardia or pauses with symptoms. A 24-hour ambulatory

Table 3.1   Indications for Pacing in Sinus Node Dysfunction

Class	Indication
I	Sinus node dysfunction with documented symptomatic bradycardia, including frequent sinus pauses that produce symptoms
I	Symptomatic chronotropic incompetence
I	Symptomatic sinus bradycardia that results from required drug therapy for medical conditions
IIa	Sinus node dysfunction with heart rate less than 40 bpm when a clear association between significant symptoms consistent with bradycardia and the actual presence of bradycardia has not been documented
IIa	Permanent pacemaker implantation is reasonable for syncope of unexplained origin when clinically significant abnormalities of sinus node function are discovered or provoked in electrophysiological studies

Adapted with permission from Epstein AE et al., ACC/AHA/HRS 2008 Guidelines for Device-Based Therapy of Cardiac Rhythm Abnormalities: Executive Summary. *Heart Rhythm*. 2008;5:934–55.

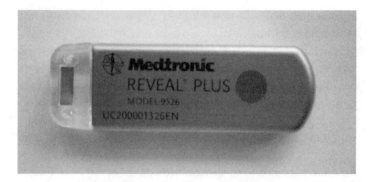

■ **Figure 3.1   Insertable loop recorder for documentation of arrhythmias in patients with syncope or other severe symptoms**

It is implanted in an infra-clavicular pocket, with no need for leads. The electrodes for recording rhythm are on the generator itself.

(Holter) monitor is typically used to determine the range of heart rates during daily activities and at night, with a diary kept by the patient to record symptoms. A continuous loop event monitor or a handheld event monitor can be used to correlate more infrequent symptoms with the cardiac rhythm. Electrophysiologic studies are almost never performed solely for evaluation of sinus node function, although they may be indicated in patients with unexplained syncope. In such cases, the evaluation includes measurement of sinus node recovery times; markedly prolonged recovery times may indicate that sinus node dysfunction is the cause of syncope. When all these modalities have been unable to determine the cardiac rhythm during symptomatic periods, insertable loop recorders may be implanted (**Figure 3.1**). They serve as automatic event recorders for periods of over a year, allowing the detection of arrhythmias associated with rare symptomatic events. Symptomatic sinus node dysfunction is a class I indication for permanent pacing.

The most useful approach to determine whether a patient with suspected sinus node dysfunction requires permanent pacing is ECG monitoring for correlation of the cardiac rhythm with symptoms. Depending on the frequency and severity of symptoms, 24-hour Holter monitoring or various types of event monitors may be most appropriate.

AV Block

Broadly speaking, AV block refers to block at any level of the AV conduction system, from the AV node through the His-Purkinje system (see Figure 2.3). AV block can be subcategorized into first-, second-, and third-degree AV block. The definition of first-degree AV block is a PR interval greater than 200 msec, with a consistent one-to-one relationship between atrial and ventricular activation. First-degree AV block by itself is not an indication for pacing, unless it is marked and itself leads to symptoms consistent with pacemaker syndrome. The latter refers to a condition in which patients have a variety of symptoms such as dizziness, fatigue, weakness, presyncope, syncope, and heart failure that are due to loss of AV synchrony. Most commonly, ventricular pacing in the setting of intact sinus node function is responsible, such as is the case with temporary ventricular pacing in a hospitalized patient. Extreme first-degree AV block can sometimes lead to similar symptoms, because atrial systole occurs right after ventricular systole and leads to the same hemodynamic consequences.

Pacemaker syndrome is a condition in which loss of AV synchrony associated with ventricular pacing leads to a variety of symptoms such as dizziness, fatigue, weakness, presyncope, syncope, and heart failure. Pacemaker syndrome can also occur in some patients with marked first-degree AV block, because the timing of atrial and ventricular systole leads to the same adverse hemodynamic consequences.

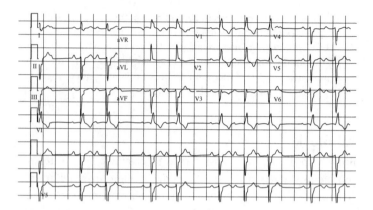

■ **Figure 3.2   ECG of Wenckebach AV block**

Note the gradual increase in PR interval before the dropped beat occurs.

Second-degree AV block is the most complicated to under-stand, but at its most basic level, it means that some but not all of the sinus node impulses reach the ventricles. There are two typical patterns of second-degree AV block seen on monitoring. The key discriminator is whether the PR interval gradually increases before an impulse to the ventricles is blocked, or whether it appears to be fixed until a dropped beat occurs. Mobitz type I (Wenckebach) AV block is the pattern characterized by a gradual increase in the PR interval until a blocked beat occurs, after which conduction resumes (**Figure 3.2**). The majority of the time, Wenckebach AV block is caused by block of conduction in the AV node itself. Occasionally, it may be due to conduction slowing in the His-Purkinje system. The QRS is narrow in most patients. If bundle branch block is present as well, the level of block is most likely in the His-Purkinje system. Regardless, Wenckebach AV block is con-sidered a class I indication for pacing in the presence of symp-toms. Typical symptoms would include exercise intolerance, fatigue, dizziness, and syncope. Younger patients and particularly well-trained athletes with chronic Mobitz type I, second-degree

AV block have a benign prognosis in the absence of structural heart disease and do not need pacing except in the presence of symptoms. It has been found that patients older than 45 years with Mobitz type I, second-degree AV block do worse in follow-up than age- and sex-matched controls, except if permanent pacemakers are in place. However, the current ACC/AHA/HRS guidelines still consider this a class III indication for pacing (i.e., not indicated). Such patients should be followed closely for the development of symptoms, to allow for timely intervention with permanent pacing if they become manifest.

Mobitz type II AV block is characterized by a fixed PR interval before a dropped beat occurs. It is caused by conduction delay in the His-Purkinje system rather than the AV node. Because it is often associated with unpredictable progression to complete AV block, permanent pacing is indicated. Given the location of the conduction block, there is often bundle branch block or an intraventricular conduction delay associated with it.

The distinction between Mobitz type I and II AV block is mainly based on whether there is a fixed PR interval before a dropped beat, or a gradual increase in PR interval before block occurs. Bundle branch block will more often be associated with Mobitz type II AV block, since the level of the block is usually in the His-Purkinje system.

Either Mobitz type I or type II AV block may progress to the point that only every other cardiac impulse is conducted to the ventricles, resulting in 2:1 AV block (**Figure 3.3**). Because there is no series of PR intervals to analyze for fixed or progressive prolongation, one cannot be sure where the location of the block is in these circumstances. If there is bundle branch block present as well, this finding provides circumstantial evidence that the level of the block is lower in the AV conduction system.

High-grade AV block is a more advanced form of second-degree AV block, with multiple nonconducted P waves. Finally,

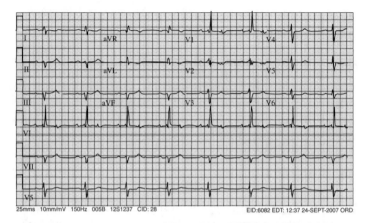

■ **Figure 3.3** An example of 2:1 AV block, with right bundle branch block and left anterior fascicular block (trifascicular block)

complete or third-degree AV block is present when no atrial impulses reach the ventricle. Third-degree AV block may be acquired, congenital, or iatrogenic, after cardiac surgery or deliberate ablation of the AV node for management of certain arrhythmias. Acquired AV block may be caused by a variety of conditions, such as progressive fibrosis in the conduction system, infiltrative diseases such as sarcoidosis or amyloidosis, myocardial infarction, certain neuromuscular diseases, infections such as Lyme disease, connective tissue diseases, and cardiomyopathies.

Class I and IIa indications for pacing in patients with advanced second-degree AV block or third-degree AV block are summarized in **Table 3.2**.

In the past, congenital complete AV block was not considered to require pacing, unless there were associated symptoms due to the bradycardia, ventricular dysfunction, complex ventricular ectopy, or a wide QRS escape rhythm. It has more recently been found that such patients are at risk for sudden cardiac death as adults. This finding has resulted in a lower threshold for recommending pacemaker implantation in such patients. Congenital

Table 3.2   Indications for Pacing in Acquired AV Block

CLASS	INDICATION
I	Third-degree and advanced second-degree AV block at any anatomic level associated with: • bradycardia with symptoms (including heart failure) or ventricular arrhythmias presumed to be due to AV block, • arrhythmias and other medical conditions that require drug therapy that results in symptomatic bradycardia, • documented periods of asystole greater than or equal to 3.0 seconds or any escape rate less than 40 bpm, or with an escape rhythm that is below the AV node, and • AF and bradycardia with 1 or more pauses of at least 5 seconds or longer.
I	After catheter ablation of the AV junction.
I	Third-degree and advanced second-degree postoperative AV block that is not expected to resolve after cardiac surgery.
I	Third-degree and advanced second-degree AV block at any anatomic level associated with neuromuscular diseases with AV block (e.g., myotonic muscular dystrophy), with or without symptoms.
I	Second-degree AV block with associated symptomatic bradycardia regardless of type or site of block.
I	Persistent third-degree AV block at any anatomic site with average awake ventricular rates of 40 bpm or faster if cardiomegaly or left ventricular dysfunction is present or if the site of block is below the AV node.
I	Second- or third-degree AV block during exercise in the absence of myocardial ischemia.
IIa	Persistent third-degree AV block with an escape rate greater than 40 bpm in asymptomatic adult patients without cardiomegaly.
IIa	Asymptomatic second-degree AV block at intra- or infra-His levels found at electrophysiological study.
IIa	First- or second-degree AV block with symptoms similar to those of pacemaker syndrome or hemodynamic compromise.
IIa	Asymptomatic type II second-degree AV block with a narrow QRS. With a wide QRS, it is a Class I recommendation.

Adapted with permission from Epstein AE et al., ACC/AHA/HRS 2008 Guidelines for Device-Based Therapy of Cardiac Rhythm Abnormalities: Executive Summary. *Heart Rhythm.* 2008;5:934–55.

complete AV block is now considered a class IIa indication for permanent pacing if patients are asymptomatic and have an adequate ventricular rate and a narrow QRS. In children and adolescents, it is still a class IIb recommendation for pacing.

> **In certain circumstances, pacing may be indicated even if a patient has not manifested symptoms, such as in many cases of third-degree AV block or Mobitz type II AV block.**

Bundle Branch Block

Isolated block in the left or right bundle branch is not an indication for pacing. The left bundle branch itself has two fascicles: anterior and posterior. Complete block in the bundle branches results in characteristic patterns on the ECG. Block in the left anterior or posterior fascicle leads to a change in the axis of the QRS on the ECG. While left bundle branch block (LBBB) itself is a form of bifascicular block, the term is usually used to refer to right bundle branch block (RBBB) in conjunction with either left anterior or posterior fascicular block. In addition to these findings, first-degree AV block is present as well in patients with trifascicular block. Patients with bundle branch block who are asymptomatic do not need further evaluation except for periodic ECGs; on the other hand, individuals with syncope require further evaluation. Many of these patients have structural heart disease. If the cause of syncope is not identified after a complete clinical evaluation, electrophysiologic testing may be indicated. The goals of such a study are not only to evaluate the AV conduction system, but also to evaluate sinus node function and inducibility of arrhythmias, both supraventricular and ventricular, potentially responsible for syncope. Findings at electrophysiologic study that would result in a class IIa indication for pacing include a markedly prolonged HV interval (>100 msec, normal being 35–55 msec) or infra-Hisian block induced with atrial pacing at a rate under 130 beats per minute. Otherwise, pacing is indicated in patients with bifascicular or trifascicular block if there is an intermittent third-degree AV block, Mobitz type II second-degree AV block, alternating bundle branch block, or syncope when other potential causes such as ventricular tachycardia (VT) have been excluded.

> **Bundle branch block by itself is not an indication for pacing. However, if a patient has symptoms such as syncope, further investigation is warranted to determine whether AV block or arrhythmias such as VT are responsible for the symptoms, because many of these patients have structural heart disease.**

Post-Myocardial Infarction

Patients who have suffered an acute myocardial infarction may develop AV conduction disturbances. Temporary pacing may be needed for symptomatic AV block or even asymptomatic advanced AV block (third-degree AV block, Mobitz type II second-degree AV block, new bilateral bundle branch block). However, the need for temporary pacing does not necessarily indicate that patients will need permanent pacing. The site of infarction in patients with AV block and a narrow QRS is usually inferior. It is typically due to reversible ischemia in the area supplied by the AV nodal artery, with the site of the block in the AV node. In most cases, the AV block will resolve, but it may take days to do so. Patients with bundle branch block and AV block most often have anterior infarctions. There is usually extensive necrosis in the septum, the site of the block is usually infranodal, and progression to complete heart block may be sudden (**Table 3.3**).

Class I indications for permanent pacing after an acute myocardial infarction include persistent, symptomatic second- or third-degree AV block. Permanent pacing is also indicated in asymptomatic transient or persistent second- or third-degree AV block with infranodal block and bundle branch block. The development of bundle branch

Table 3.3   AV Block in Acute Myocardial Infarction

CHARACTERISTIC	ANTERIOR MI	INFERIOR MI
Pathophysiology	Necrosis of septum	Ischemia involving AV nodal artery
Site of block	His-Purkinje system	AV node
Intraventricular conduction delay	Common	Rare
Progression to complete AV block	Sudden	Gradual
Escape rhythm	Ventricular	Junctional

AV=atrioventricular; MI=myocardial infarction

block and advanced AV block in the setting of an acute myocardial infarction is good evidence that the level of block is infranodal. If there is doubt as to the level of block, it is possible to do an electrophysiologic study to determine whether the block is intra- or infranodal. However, an electrophysiologic study is rarely necessary today, because most such patients will have poor ventricular function due to extensive infarction. These patients will thus be candidates for implantable cardioverter defibrillators (ICDs), which have built-in pacemakers, for primary prevention of sudden cardiac death. However, it is important to remember that, in making decisions about the timing of implantation and the type of device to implant, current Medicare guidelines stipulate that ICDs should not be implanted within 40 days of an acute myocardial infarction.

Heart Failure and Dyssynchrony

Patients with symptomatic heart failure may have intra- and interventricular dyssynchrony that contributes to ventricular dysfunction. Early attempts to use pacing to improve heart failure depended on right ventricular pacing with short programmed AV delays. While the initial reports were favorable, the results were not reproducible, and it has subsequently been recognized that chronic right ventricular pacing alone can actually be deleterious. Subsequent investigations used biventricular pacing, with a lead in a lateral or posterolateral branch of the CS for left ventricular pacing as well as a lead in the right ventricle. Such CRT has been demonstrated to result in improvement in the New York Heart Association (NYHA) classification of heart failure symptoms, quality of life, and exercise tolerance in the majority of patients. Reverse ventricular remodeling (reduction in ventricular chamber size and improvement in left ventricular ejection fraction [LVEF]) as well as improvement in survival have also been demonstrated.

Most patients with ventricular dyssynchrony have LBBB or a marked intraventricular conduction delay. The recently revised device guidelines categorize patients with class III and ambulatory class IV heart failure that is refractory to medical therapy who have sinus rhythm, a QRS duration ≥120 msec, and LVEF ≤ 35 percent as having a class I indication for CRT. For patients with AF, it is considered a class IIa indication for CRT. It is also a class IIa indication for CRT when patients have systolic heart failure and frequent dependence on ventricular pacing. Although QRS duration alone is a rather crude indication of dyssynchrony, recent studies have not shown echocardiography to be superior in identifying candidates most likely to respond to CRT. Patients with advanced class IV symptoms should be carefully considered as to whether they are appropriate candidates for CRT, because prognosis is usually poor for these patients even with intervention. There are ongoing clinical trials evaluating the use of CRT in other patient populations, such as those with class II heart failure symptoms or those with AV block requiring pacing, to see if CRT can retard the progression of heart failure. However, one recent trial, REVERSE (Resynchronization Reverses Remodeling in Systolic Left Ventricular Dysfunction), did not show a significant improvement in outcome with CRT in patients with class II heart failure symptoms.

> Candidates for CRT include patients with NYHA class III–IV
> heart failure refractory to medical therapy, LVEF ≤ 35%,
> and QRS duration ≥ 120 msec.

Hypersensitive Carotid Sinus Syndrome

Hypersensitive carotid sinus syndrome is a condition whereby patients have extreme sensitivity to carotid sinus stimulation. There may be primarily a cardioinhibitory response, with asystole due to sinus arrest or AV block lasting at least 3 seconds, a vasodepressor response with hypotension, or a mixed response. Characteristically, patients may have presyncope or syncope with sudden and extreme head positioning, such as reaching up to get something off a high shelf. Carotid sinus massage is used with ECG monitoring to elicit the cardioinhibitory response. It should be emphasized that patients, particularly the elderly, may have hypersensitive carotid sinus responses but not the true syndrome with associated syncope. Thus, it is important to correlate symptoms with the cardioinhibitory response before considering pacemaker implantation, especially since pacemakers cannot correct the vasodepressor component.

Neurocardiogenic Syncope

Neurocardiogenic syncope refers to a syndrome in which activation of a neural reflex leads to systemic hypotension with bradycardia and peripheral vasodilation. Episodes may be triggered by pain, stress, or anxiety and typically occur in patients with structurally normal hearts. It is rather common in adolescents and young adults. Management may include recognition of prodromal symptoms and taking measures to prevent or abort the episodes (staying well hydrated, lying down with the feet elevated if symptoms develop), a variety of medications, and pacing in a small minority of patients. The role of pacing in this condition has been controversial. As with hypersensitive carotid sinus syndrome, the vasodepressor component may predominate in some patients, rendering pacing ineffective in controlling symptoms. Dual-chamber pacing is now considered only a class IIb indication for pacing in selected patients with recurrent, significant symptoms and documented severe bradycardia or asystole. If pacing is used, a generator with rate-drop response should be considered. Rate-drop response is a feature whereby a sudden drop in heart rate elicits a higher pacing rate for a limited period of time (minutes), followed by a gradual return to the baseline pacing rate.

Hypertrophic Cardiomyopathy

There was great interest at one time in the use of dual-chamber pacemakers for the management of patients with hypertrophic cardiomyopathy. Early nonrandomized studies showed a reduction in left ventricular outflow tract gradient with dual-chamber pacing with a short AV delay. However, randomized trials failed to show an improvement in quality of life, and there was a significant placebo effect demonstrated. Currently, there are no data that demonstrate that pacing alters the clinical course of patients with hypertrophic cardiomyopathy. Therefore, hypertrophic cardiomyopathy is no better than a class IIb indication for pacing. Patients who are highly symptomatic with significant outflow tract gradients should be considered for septal myectomy or alcohol septal ablation in preference to pacing.

Long QT Syndrome

Initial treatment of patients with congenital long QT syndrome associated with symptomatic ventricular arrhythmias is usually beta blockade. If symptoms persist, permanent pacing may be considered, particularly if ventricular arrhythmias are pause dependent or related to bradycardia. However, because the major concern in such patients is sudden cardiac death from ventricular arrhythmias, a dual-chamber ICD will often be implanted if the decision is made to go with device therapy.

Sleep Apnea

Patients with sleep apnea are at increased risk for hypertension, bradyarrhythmias, AF, and exacerbation of heart failure. There have been several studies demonstrating improvement in sleep apnea after patients have received pacemakers for standard indications, such as sinus node dysfunction and AV block. Observational studies have shown that dual-chamber pacing is superior to ventricular pacing alone in this circumstance. However, randomized studies to date have not shown an improvement in hypopnea/apnea episodes with pacing. Thus, pacing should only be employed in these patients at the present time if there is an independent, standard indication for pacing.

Cardiac Transplantation

Bradyarrhythmias are fairly common after cardiac transplantation. Because of vagal denervation in the transplanted heart, resting heart rates are expected to be higher than in normal hearts. Significant bradycardia and asystole have been associated with sudden cardiac death in follow-up. However, sinus bradycardia in transplanted patients often resolves in the first 6 to 12 months. Pacing should be considered in transplant patients based on standard indications, or if there is significant bradycardia that is not expected to resolve.

Suggested Readings

Epstein AE, DiMarco JP, Ellenbogen KA, et al. ACC/AHA/HRS 2008 Guidelines for Device-Based Therapy of Cardiac Rhythm Abnormalities: Executive Summary. *Heart Rhythm.* 2008;5:934–955.

Krahn AD, Klein GJ, Skanes AC, et al. Use of the implantable loop recorder in evaluation of patients with unexplained syncope. *J Cardiovasc Electrophysiol.* 2003;14(9 Suppl):S70–73.

Lamas GA, Lee KL, Sweeney MO, et al. Mode Selection Trial in sinus node dysfunction: Ventricular pacing or dual chamber pacing for sinus node dysfunction. *N Engl J Med.* 2002;346:1854–1862.

4 ■ Leads

Pacemaker leads are insulated wires with one or more electrodes at the distal end and a connector at the proximal end. The electrode is positioned in the heart in the chamber to be paced, and the connector attaches the lead to the pacemaker generator. The purpose of these leads is twofold: first, to allow sensing of cardiac electrical signals from a particular chamber of the heart and deliver that information to the generator; and second, to deliver pacing impulses from the generator to the myocardium.

Lead Design

A pacing lead is comprised of an electrode, conductor, insulation, and a connector (**Figure 4.1**). The electrode at the tip of a pacing lead may be made of a variety of materials, mostly including platinum (platinum, platinum-iridium, platinum coated with titanium) or titanium (titanium, titanium oxide, titanium alloys, iridium oxide-coated titanium, titanium nitride). The small size of the electrode tip of modern pacing leads results in a high current density and low pacing stimulation threshold, which help to lessen current drain on the battery. A textured or porous design of the electrode tip provides the added advantage of low polarization without affecting stimulation threshold. Polarization refers to the fact that ions can build up over time at the tip of the lead, making it more difficult to pace the heart.

A pacemaker lead must have a conductor to transmit signals bidirectionally between the heart and the generator. The conductor needs to be flexible and resistant to metal fatigue. A typical conductor material is MP35N, which is an alloy of nickel, chromium, cobalt, and molybdenum that is highly corrosion resistant. Often a central core of a highly conductive material such as silver is used that is surrounded by MP35N using techniques known as drawn brazen strand (DBS) or drawn filled tube (DFT).

Insulation is required on the conductor to prevent leakage of current into the bloodstream before it reaches the tip of the lead

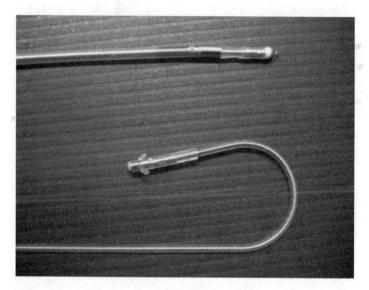

■ Figure 4.1   Unipolar and bipolar pacing leads

On top is shown a bipolar lead with a fixed screw. There is a ring electrode proximal to the tip. On the bottom is shown a unipolar, passive fixation, atrial J lead. There is no ring electrode. The J shape allows stable positioning of the lead in the RAA.

Courtesy of Boston Scientific, Inc.

and the myocardium. Insulation also separates one conductor from the other in the case of bipolar leads. The most common types of insulation are silicone and polyurethane. There is a longer history of silicone use as an insulator, and it is a highly durable type of insulation. However, silicone nicks and abrades easily, and it has a high coefficient of friction. The latter can make it more difficult to manipulate leads independently when two silicone leads are placed through the same access site. In order to counteract this problem, some silicone leads have special coatings to help make them more lubricious.

Polyurethane leads are a more recent development, but even they have been available for many years. Different polyurethane polymers have been developed for permanent transvenous leads.

Some types have had a problem in the past with early deterioration of the insulation and are no longer marketed. Current polyurethane leads have proven to be quite reliable. Their "slicker" surface makes it a little easier to manipulate adjacent leads independently. However, regardless of the type of lead insulation, there always may be some difficulty manipulating leads independently when a single access site has been used. Finally, there are silicone-polyurethane hybrids that have been developed for use in pacing leads. They are designed to provide the flexibility of high-performance silicone rubber with the strength, tear resistance, and abrasion resistance of polyurethane.

Whatever the lead design, there must be a means to connect the lead to the pacemaker generator. Different sizes and shapes of connectors along with differences in the connector blocks of pacemaker generators made it difficult early on to attach some leads to new generators, necessitating the use of adaptors in some instances. Adaptors should be avoided if at all possible, because any extra hardware adds bulk to the pacemaker pocket and also increases the chances of a loose connection or breakdown that can lead to failure to deliver pacing therapy. For these reasons, industry-wide standards have been adopted for pacemaker leads. The typical pacemaker lead has what is called an IS-1 connector ("Industry Standard," 3.2 mm pin). Any lead with an IS-1 connector will fit into any pacemaker generator, including those of other manufacturers, with IS-1 connector blocks. Extremely old pacing leads may still have 5 or 6 mm connectors that are not IS-1 compatible. If they are working properly, there is no need to replace them, but either a generator will need to be used that accepts such a lead, or an adaptor will be necessary.

A pacing lead is comprised of an electrode, conductor, insulation, and a connector. Unipolar leads have a single electrode and conductor, while bipolar leads have two of each that are electrically isolated by the insulation.

Bipolar and Unipolar Leads

Cardiac pacing leads may be either bipolar or unipolar. When transvenous leads were first developed, unipolar leads were the only kind available. Even when the first bipolar leads were developed, their larger diameter led many physicians to continue to prefer unipolar leads. Advances in lead design have been such that bipolar leads have a profile as small as or smaller than old unipolar leads. Today, unipolar leads are almost nonexistent in transvenous applications.

The differences in design of a unipolar lead compared to a bipolar lead can be seen in Figure 4.1. A unipolar lead has a single electrode at the tip of the lead. Because current flow requires a closed circuit, in a unipolar system, current flows from the tip of the lead through the myocardium and the chest up to the pacemaker generator, which constitutes the other end of the circuit. The relatively large circuit leads to a large pacing artifact on the ECG (**Figure 4.2**). In addition, the inclusion of the pectoralis muscle and other structures between the tip of the lead and the generator makes unipolar pacing prone to the problem of myopotential inhibition and electromagnetic interference (EMI); that is, tremor or twitching of the muscles of the chest may create enough of a signal as detected by the pacing lead to lead to inhibition of pacing, a known disadvantage of unipolar pacing.

With bipolar pacing, the electrode at the tip of the pacing lead is similar to that found with unipolar pacing. There is a second conductor wire in a bipolar lead, with insulation separating the two conductors from each other and also separating the conductors from the bloodstream. There are a couple of different designs for bipolar leads. They may be coaxial, in that the inner conductor is covered by the first layer of insulation, which is surrounded by the second conductor, which then is covered by the outer insulation. An alternative design is for each conductor to be covered by insulation, with each conductor coil wound together in a "coradial" design, with an outer insulation covering. One advantage of

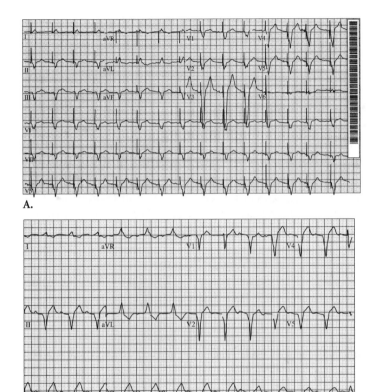

A.

B.

■ **Figure 4.2   Pacing artifact on ECG**

A. Unipolar pacing.

B. Bipolar pacing. Note the much smaller artifact with bipolar pacing.

coradial leads is that they can be manufactured in a thinner size compared to coaxial leads.

In addition to the second conductor, bipolar pacing leads have a ring about a centimeter proximal to the tip of the lead. The tip and the ring may be covered with iridium oxide, which promotes low chronic pacing thresholds. During bipolar pacing, current flows from the tip of the lead to the ring. This is a much smaller circuit than with unipolar pacing, leading to a very small pacing artifact on the ECG and much less risk of myopotential inhibition (see Figure 4.2). With the small profile and reliability of modern bipolar pacing leads, there is rarely a reason to use unipolar leads for permanent transvenous pacing in the right atrium or right ventricle. Unipolar leads still have a place in left ventricular pacing, because the small size permits placement in small branches of the CS. It should be noted that most pacemaker generators will permit bipolar leads to be programmed unipolar, if there is some advantage to be had (such as early insulation failure in a bipolar lead before definitive correction of the problem can be undertaken).

Fixation: Active Versus Passive

Pacing leads must be attached to the myocardium by some means to allow stable sensing and pacing. Transvenous leads are placed in the heart either by passive or active fixation. Passive fixation leads have either tines or fins (tines being most common today) near the lead tip (**Figure 4.3A**). These tines become caught up in the trabeculations of the right ventricle, or alternatively, in the RAA, and then maintain their position in the heart until fibrosis develops that holds the lead in place more firmly. Passive fixation leads exhibit higher dislodgement rates than active fixation leads, and for this reason, they are less often used in pacemaker-dependent patients.

Active fixation leads have a screw at the tip of the lead that is advanced into the myocardium at the time of implantation. The screw may be electrically inert, in which case there must be a separate electrode at the tip, or electrically active. In some lead designs, the tip is fixed and exposed at the end of the lead (**Figure 4.3B**). In order to allow atraumatic introduction of the lead into the heart, a sugar coating (mannitol) is placed over the screw during the manufacturing process. This sugar coating naturally dissolves in the

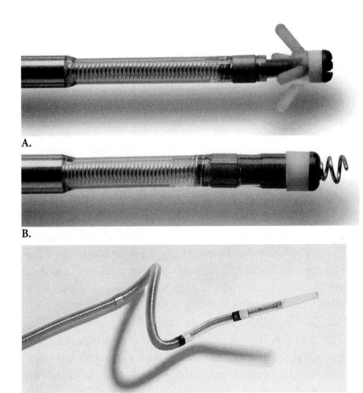

A.

B.

C.

■ Figure 4.3   Types of fixation

A. Passive fixation pacing lead.

B. Active fixation lead with a fixed screw.

C. CS lead.

Courtesy of Boston Scientific, Inc.

heart once the lead is placed in the vascular system, exposing the screw. The lead is then fixed in the heart by rotating the lead body with the tip against the myocardium, advancing the screw into the tissue. The disadvantage of this type of lead is that once the mannitol dissolves, the exposed screw can get caught up in the valves and other locations where they are not meant to be fixed. Another type of fixed screw lead is a thin 4.1 Fr bipolar active fixation lead with no lumen that is delivered to the desired location by a steerable catheter. The lead can thus be fixed in very specific locations, such as Bachmann's bundle.

The alternative and more common active fixation lead design today involves an extendable and retractable screw. With this type of lead, there is no exposed screw as the lead is advanced through the vascular system. Once the lead is in the desired location in the heart, the screw is advanced by means of a fixation tool that rotates the pin at the proximal end of the lead that is directly connected to and advances the screw at the distal end of the lead. The screw may be electrically active or inert. While passive fixation leads must be placed in locations that will naturally hold the lead in place (right ventricular apex [RVA], RAA), active fixation leads may be placed in any alternative desired location, such as Bachmann's bundle or the right ventricular septum.

The choice of an active or a passive fixation lead is, to a large extent, simply the preference of the physician implanting the lead. There are certain considerations, however, that may impact which type of lead is chosen in an individual situation. For example, patients with moderate or severe tricuspid regurgitation would be better served by the use of an active fixation lead in the ventricle. It can be quite challenging in these patients to advance the lead across the tricuspid valve and position the lead adequately. The active fixation minimizes the chances of lead dislodgement. In the atrium, active fixation leads are often chosen in patients who have previously undergone cardiac surgery, because the atrial appendage may have been amputated at the time of surgery or otherwise not have an optimal shape to hold a passive fixation lead in place. Another advantage of active fixation leads is their low profile; that is, the lead tip is the same diameter as the lead body. In the event that a lead needs extraction at a later date, the low profile may make extraction of the lead tip from the heart a little easier technically.

On the other hand, perforation, particularly of the thin-walled atrium, is more likely with an active fixation lead. Although this is unlikely to lead to tamponade, pericarditis may occur in rare situations from the exposed screw irritating the pericardium. Before the widespread use of steroid-eluting leads (noted later), another disadvantage of active fixation leads was a higher incidence of exit block. Exit block occurs when a lead fibroses into the heart to such an extent that the inert scar prevents adequate pacing. Sensing is usually adequate, but pacing thresholds can rise to the point of inability to capture the heart. The trauma associated with active fixation makes exit block more likely than with passive fixation leads. Fortunately, the use of steroid-eluting leads has nearly eliminated this problem.

A final consideration regarding active versus passive fixation occurs when a lead needs to be repositioned in the heart during the implantation procedure. If the lead can be secured in the right atrium or ventricle on the first attempt and sensing, pacing threshold, and impedance are adequate (see Chapter 6), either a passive or active fixation lead is acceptable. However, there are often situations in which sensing and/or pacing is poor in a particular location and multiple attempts at repositioning the lead are necessary. With a passive fixation lead, there are limited locations where the lead can be placed if the initial position is not adequate, because the leads were specifically designed for the appendage or the apex. On the other hand, although an active fixation lead can be positioned in alternative locations, multiple attempts at advancing and retracting the screw may lead to tissue getting caught up in the fixation mechanism. Ultimately, it may become impossible to fix the lead to the myocardium adequately and the lead may need to be abandoned. This problem may be particularly evident in patients with severe right atrial or right ventricular dilatation. In either case, the passive or active fixation lead may need to be replaced by a new active fixation lead in order to achieve adequate positioning in the heart.

Passive fixation leads have tines or fins to stabilize them in the heart. Active fixation leads have either a fixed or an extendable-retractable screw.

Steroid Elution

Whether there are tines or a screw at the end of a pacing lead for fixation in the heart, there is some degree of injury to the adjacent myocardium that occurs naturally at the time of lead implantation. Over the initial weeks after pacemaker implantation, the inflammation resolves and fibrosis forms at the tip of the lead. The scar tissue makes late lead dislodgement highly unlikely. However, the fibrosis can also cause pacing thresholds to rise, sometimes to unacceptable levels. To counteract this problem, steroid-eluting leads have been developed. These leads release minute amounts of dexamethasone sodium phosphate or acetate from the tip of the lead over a period of time. The steroid tends to reduce inflammation and leads to lower chronic pacing thresholds than with standard leads. Such leads are now commonly used clinically because of their distinct advantages and lack of identified disadvantages. In passive fixation leads, a silicone rubber plug compounded with <1 mg dexamethasone is placed in an internal chamber immediately behind a porous electrode, and it communicates with the outer surface of the electrode through a porous chamber. In active fixation leads, a porous silicone rubber collar impregnated with dexamethasone is positioned around the tip electrode.

Steroid-eluting leads are used in almost all pacing applications today because they result in lower chronic pacing thresholds.

Design Features for Implantation in Different Cardiac Chambers

Right Atrium

Leads placed in the right atrium are usually placed in the atrial appendage. With passive fixation leads, this is far and away the most stable location for the lead. The distal end of the lead has a "J" shape to it. A stylet is positioned in the lumen of the lead to straighten it out as it is advanced into the right atrium. When the lead is in the mid- to low-right atrium, the stylet is pulled back, allowing the lead to resume its natural J shape. The J shape hooks up into the RAA in an anteromedial position. If the RAA is distorted or amputated, as may occur after cardiac surgery, passive fixation leads may not maintain a stable position. In such cases, use of an active fixation lead is preferable.

Active fixation leads designed for use in the atrium may have a fixed J at the distal end or, more commonly, they may be straight leads (see Figure 4.1). The latter are fixed in position using a J stylet, so that attachment of the lead in the atrial appendage is possible. As a matter of fact, the only difference between straight active fixation leads used in the atrium versus those used in the ventricle is the length of the lead, with shorter leads employed in the atrium so that there is less redundant lead in the pacemaker pocket. Shorter leads may also be chosen when the pacemaker is placed on the right side of the chest, because there is a shorter distance to the heart.

While active fixation leads are most often placed in the RAA, the active fixation mechanism permits placement of the lead in any stable location in the right atrium. There has been some interest in placing leads in the septum or Bachmann's bundle (a band of tissue connecting the right and the left atrium that facilitates rapid interatrial conduction of electrical impulses). These alternative locations have been promoted as superior locations for atrial pacing leads because of more rapid and physiologic conduction of impulses through the atria. However, there is no uniform consensus at the present time that routine placement of atrial leads in these alternative locations is necessary or desirable.

Given the thin atrial wall, it is possible that the screw of the pacing lead may extend beyond the epicardium in some patients, particularly with a more lateral or posterior lead position. While tamponade is rare, as is pericarditis from direct irritation of the lead on the pericardium, it is better to avoid the lateral atrial wall unless there is no alternative stable position.

With leads placed in the RAA, active fixation allows the operator to leave a little more slack in the lead than with a passive fixation lead, because the active fixation should result in a minimal risk of dislodgement with change in the patient's position after implantation.

Right atrial leads are usually placed in the appendage, although alternative locations may be selected if an active fixation lead is used. It is advisable to avoid locations low in the atrium, in order to minimize the risk of far-field sensing of R waves.

Right Ventricle

Leads that are meant to be placed in the RVA are straight. Whether an active or a passive fixation lead is selected, a curved stylet is used to advance the lead to the right ventricular outflow tract (see Chapter 6). This stylet is exchanged for a straight stylet that will cause the lead to fall naturally toward the apex as it is pulled back, after which the lead can be advanced gently to a stable location. If an alternative location is desired for the right ventricular lead, such as septal placement, use of an active fixation lead is mandatory. The amount of slack that is left in a lead placed in the right ventricle is the same whether the lead is an active or a passive fixation lead.

Left Ventricle (Coronary Sinus)

There is a different set of challenges for leads placed in the CS for left ventricular pacing. Given that the lead sits in the CS, it is not possible to fix it in place with a screw. Early designs for these leads had a simple curve or an "S" shape at the distal end of the lead; in some cases, there were small tines near the tip. With a stylet or guide wire advanced to the end of the lead, the curve would be straightened out, but when it was removed, the curvature would be restored. The curve or "S" allows the lead to brace itself against the walls of the vein in which it is placed (see Figure 4.3C).

The more common type of lead design today has an open tip as well as a lumen, so that the lead can accept either a stylet or, alternatively, a guide wire that may be advanced through the distal end of the lead. The advantage of this design is that the guide wire may be easier to advance into the desired branch of the CS, after which the lead itself is advanced over the guide wire and the latter is removed. These over-the-wire (OTW) leads may either be unipolar or bipolar.

There is an alternative bipolar lead design with a larger and more rigid tip. Although this lead does not have an open lumen at the tip for use with a guide wire, the shape may be an advantage when placing leads in large branches of the CS. In such cases, small caliber OTW leads may not anchor securely in the CS and may be more prone to dislodgement. In any case, the lack of a true fixation mechanism at the tip of any of these leads makes them more prone to dislodgement than leads placed in the right atrium or ventricle.

The most common type of lead used in the CS is an OTW lead that uses a guide wire for subselection of the branch for placement of the lead. The inability to fix the lead securely in the CS leads to a higher rate of dislodgement of these leads compared to right atrial or right ventricular leads.

Epicardial Leads

Most leads are placed transvenously, but pacing leads may be placed epicardially as well. Often this is done at the time of cardiac surgery for other reasons, but it may be done as a primary procedure through a thoracotomy. Reasons for the use of epicardial leads may include lack of venous access because of occlusion, mechanical tricuspid valve replacement, a history of endocarditis, or certain types of congenital heart disease. Various types of fixation mechanisms have been used for epicardial leads, mostly involving hooks or screws. Epicardial pacing thresholds tend to be higher than transvenous thresholds. Recently, steroid-eluting epicardial leads have become available that have a porous platinum button-shaped configuration that can be used in a bipolar configuration.

Suggested Readings

Ellenbogen KA, Wood MA, Gilligan DM, et al. Steroid eluting high impedance pacing leads decrease short and long-term current drain: Results from a multicenter clinical trial. *Pacing Clin Electrophysiol.* 1999;22:39–48.

Kistler PM, Liew G, Mond HG. Long-term performance of active-fixation pacing leads: A prospective study. *Pacing Clin Electrophysiol.* 2006;29:226–230.

Sack S, Heinzel F, Dagres N, et al. Stimulation of the left ventricle through the coronary sinus with a newly developed "over the wire" lead system—early experiences with lead handling and positioning. *Europace.* 2001;3:317–323.

5 ■ Pacemaker Generator

A pacemaker generator has several different key components. It contains a battery as well as circuitry for sensing and pacing, telemetry, a microprocessor, memory, and sensors, all of which are encased in a titanium can. A pacemaker generator has a connector block for attachment of the pacing leads to the generator. Pacemaker generators today are quite small, on the order of 8–12 cc. Advances in technology have permitted this reduction in size, but counteracting this trend is the more sophisticated pacemaker functionality now present in pacemakers that requires more complex circuitry.

Battery

A number of different types of batteries for permanent pacemakers were used in the early days of pacing, one example being mercury zinc. However, technology quickly evolved toward almost exclusive use of lithium-iodine batteries. Chemical reactions at the anode and the cathode in the battery cause the conversion of lithium and iodine to lithium iodide. Lithium-iodine has several distinct advantages as an energy source in pacemakers. It provides reliable pacing over a period of many years. Its energy density is quite good, which means that the battery can be manufactured in a small size. The lack of gas produced by the chemical reaction in the battery allows for hermetic sealing of the titanium can and the header. Finally, a lithium-iodine battery has a predictable and reliable decrease in voltage as internal impedance increases near the end of its usable life, thus allowing for reasonably spaced monitoring of a patient's pacemaker and elective scheduling of replacements. There is inherently a relatively high internal impedance in lithium-iodine batteries, which is not usually a problem because the current required by pacemaker circuits is so low. To stimulate the heart with voltages that are greater than the battery voltage, circuitry with capacitors is used to double or triple the battery voltage. Capacitors are also used to reduce fluctuations in battery voltage due to the pacing pulses for all of the pacemaker circuitry.

While lithium-iodine batteries can provide low power over long periods of time, they are not ideal for providing high power over short periods of time. This makes them less suitable for high-current operations such as burst pacing and long-range telemetry. New chemistries for pacemaker batteries are being developed, including carbon monofluoride and manganese dioxide, that can provide low power over long periods of time and high power over short periods of time. These chemistries may supplant lithium-iodine as an energy source in the future pacemakers.

Advantages of lithium-iodine as an energy source in pacemaker batteries include reliability, high energy density, small size, and a predictable decrease in voltage near the end of its usable life.

A typical battery has approximately 2.8 V with an internal impedance in the hundreds of ohms at the beginning of service (BOS). It should be noted that the nomenclature for product battery life terms is changing to the new European Committee for Electrotechnical Standardization (CENELEC) standard (**Table 5.1**). The terms are all slightly different from those used in the past, and in some cases, they have different implications for patient follow-up. For example, the term ERI (elective replacement indicator) has been replaced by RRT (recommended replacement time). RRT indicates that at least 180 days remain before end of service (EOS) for at least 95 percent of pacemakers. Even though ERI is not a required battery life indicator according to the new CENELEC standard, some manufacturers choose to keep ERI as an additional indicator that approximately 90 days remain before the projected EOS.

As the RRT is reached, voltage falls to around 2.6 V and internal cell impedance increases (e.g., impedance rises to several thousand ohms for lithium-iodine batteries). Modern pacemakers are designed to provide approximately 6 months' warning

Table 5.1   Nomenclature for Product Battery Life Terms

NOMENCLATURE IN EN 45502-2-1: 2003		PREVIOUSLY USED NOMENCLATURE	
BOS	Beginning of Service	BOL	Beginning of Life
EOS	End of Service	EOL	End of Life
RRT	Recommended Replacement Time	ERI	Elective Replacement Indicator
PSP	Prolonged Service Period	Post-ERI Conditions	
Projected Service Life		Longevity	

Reproduced with permission of Medtronic, Inc.

before EOS is reached. There is no requirement for functionality changes at RRT according to the standard. Some manufacturers may choose to change magnet rates at this time. For pacemakers with ERI as a secondary indicator, pacemaker functionality may become somewhat limited, usually by pacing at a fixed rate and eliminating features such as rate response. The loss of rate response or change in pacing mode may cause a patient who is highly pacemaker dependent to develop symptoms such as exercise intolerance. Such a development is useful to bring a patient to medical attention, if for any reason routine in-office or remote follow-up has been missed. At a lower voltage around 2.0 V, the battery has reached EOS and must be replaced promptly to prevent loss of pacing from inadequate output. Even though one may tell the patient that the battery has become depleted and needs to be replaced, in fact it is the entire pacemaker generator that is replaced, because the battery and other components are hermetically sealed within the pacemaker can. An advantage to a new generator, in addition to a fresh battery, is that patients will receive the most state-of-the-art technology for their pacing indication. Battery status (BOS, RRT, or EOS) can be determined by reviewing the pacemaker interrogation, or alternatively, by analyzing the response of the pacemaker to application of a magnet (see Chapter 12).

> **Patients should be scheduled for a generator change when the RRT is evident, indicating that approximately 6 months of battery life remain. If the RRT is missed and the patient presents at EOS, generator replacement should be scheduled promptly.**

The time course over which a battery becomes depleted depends on a number of factors. There is a self-discharge of the battery even if it is still in its sterile packaging and has not been implanted in a patient. The self-discharge is due to small amounts of current that are required to keep the internal circuitry running. The longevity of a pacemaker depends more importantly on the amount of pacing that the patient requires, the programmed outputs for pacing, and the impedance of the pacing leads. A patient who is 100 percent pacemaker-dependent and has relatively high pacing thresholds and low pacing lead impedances will require a generator change much earlier than a patient with a rare need for pacing, low pacing thresholds and programmed outputs, and higher pacing lead impedance. Manufacturers provide estimates of battery longevity based on average values for these different factors, but an individual patient may have wide variations from these estimates depending on the factors just outlined.

Circuitry

Integrated Circuit

The basic building block of a pacemaker generator is an IC. An IC is a silicon wafer onto which miniaturized circuit elements are etched during manufacturing. These circuit elements are built up in layers, with millions of electronic elements. There are also discrete components in addition to ICs that are necessary for pacemaker operation, such as capacitors, diodes, inductors, and transmission coils. The ICs and discrete components are mounted onto a layered substrate (usually a flexible polymer, although

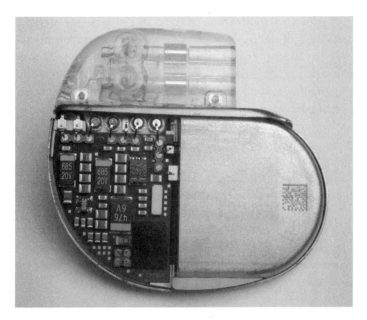

■ **Figure 5.1** **Cutaway view of a dual chamber pacemaker**

The titanium can has been partially removed to show the circuit board and the battery. On the top is the clear epoxy header, with two ports, one for the atrial lead and one for the ventricular lead.

Reproduced with permission of Medtronic, Inc.

ceramic was used in the past). The term hybrid circuit refers to the ICs plus the discrete components and the substrate on which they are mounted. Together, the hybrid circuit and the battery take up 80 to 90 percent of the space in the can (**Figure 5.1**).

> **Aside from the battery, the other major component of the pacemaker generator is the hybrid circuit, which consists of ICs, other discrete components such as capacitors and transmission coils, and the polymer on which they are mounted.**

The pacemaker generator must be able to sense the presence and timing of cardiac electrical signals and deliver outputs to pace the heart as programmed. In order to accomplish these tasks, specific circuitry is necessary (**Figure 5.2**). Sensing circuitry allows for the amplification and filtering of cardiac signals, and for the rejection of noncardiac signals (myopotentials, EMI). A sense amplifier has features such as gain, dynamic range, sensitivity, signal-to-noise ratio, and filtering capability. The sense amplifier gain allows an increase in the magnitude of the signal received from the heart to a value that can be detected and processed reliably by the rest of the circuitry. A sense amplifier also has a threshold comparator, in which a reference voltage is set that determines when an intracardiac signal is detected as a P wave or an R wave. Sensed intracardiac electrograms (EGMs) can also be displayed real time by the pacemaker programmer (for immediate review) or stored (for later review; memory intensive).

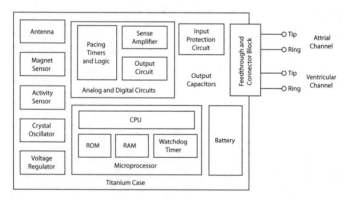

■ Figure 5.2   Block diagram of an implantable pulse generator

The circuit board, to which the battery is connected, has a microprocessor, ICs that govern pacemaker functioning, capacitors, and sensors. There is a feedthrough to the connector block where the leads are attached, so signals from the heart can be transmitted to the generator and pacing outputs delivered through the pacing leads.

Reproduced with permission of Medtronic, Inc.

Filtering is necessary to allow cardiac signals to be detected while attenuating other cardiac signals such as T waves and rejecting noncardiac signals such as myopotentials, electrical noise from the pacemaker itself, and electromechanical interference. The filters are selected on the basis of the known frequencies of intracardiac signals, with a band pass typically in the range of 20–80 Hz.

Sense amplifiers and filters in the sensing circuitry help to detect intracardiac signals while rejecting undesirable cardiac signals such as T waves and noncardiac signals such as myopotentials.

Almost all pacemakers implanted today are capable of rate-responsive pacing, and thus a sensor must be present in the hybrid circuit to allow determination of the appropriate rate of pacing. Sensors for rate-responsive pacing are covered in Chapter 8.

There is also output circuitry for the delivery of pacing pulses. Components of the output circuitry include capacitors and electrical switches controlled by the microprocessor or logic circuitry. There is also timing circuitry involved in the delivery of pacing pulses. Voltage amplifiers multiply the voltage output to deliver outputs greater than 2.8 V by means of a charge pump, which uses small capacitors to dump charge into a larger capacitor. Voltage is regulated to maintain its value as programmed as the battery voltage declines.

In addition to sensing and output, other functions of the hybrid circuit include logic and control, timing, memory, data transmission, and programming. These functions are controlled by a microprocessor, which functions much like the CPU in a computer. The microprocessor is incorporated onto the IC. The speed of the microprocessor is dependent on a crystal oscillator or clock. Inputs are received from the oscillator, sensing circuitry, and rate-responsive sensors, and the algorithms accessed from memory indicate what the response of the pacemaker should be. Memory in a pacemaker consists of read-only memory, or ROM, which is used for critical pacemaker codes, and random-access memory, or RAM. The latter can be changed throughout the life-span of the device and is used for storing programmable parameters and diagnostic information. Modern pacemakers may also include nonvolatile memory such as EEPROM (Electrically Erasable Programmable Read-Only Memory) or flash memory, which allows the pacemaker to maintain critical therapy programming in the event of a power interruption.

Telemetry

Also contained within the pacemaker generator is telemetry capability, by which bidirectional radiofrequency transmission of data and instructions is possible between the pacemaker generator and the programmer. A programmer is a specialized computer used for the interrogation of the pacemaker, so that the clinician can see how the pacemaker is working and, if necessary, adjust the settings of the pacemaker. There is dedicated circuitry to control the specifics of the communication. The peak current involved in telemetry is greater than that needed for any other function in a pacemaker, on the order of 60 μA. Long-range telemetry requires even greater current drain, on the order of several mA. Fortunately, because telemetry is used only during implantation, remote interrogation, and follow-up visits, this current drain has a negligible effect on the battery. However, the high peak currents required by telemetry do limit telemetry distance and speed.

Reed Switch

One other component of a pacemaker that should be mentioned is the reed switch. A reed switch has two thin pieces of magnetic metal that are in close proximity but do not touch each other. When a magnet is applied over the pacemaker generator, the pieces of metal do touch and thus close the electrical circuit. When a pacemaker is in "magnet mode," there is asynchronous pacing. In addition, every generator has a manufacturer- and model-specific pacing rate at BOS, RRT, and EOS when a magnet is applied. Some models allow the magnet mode to be programmed off, which may be useful for patients who cannot avoid encounters with electromagnetic fields. An alternative to the reed switch that is found in many modern pacemakers is a Hall effect sensor, which is an IC version of the mechanical reed switch.

> **A reed switch is closed by application of a magnet over the pacemaker generator, which results in most cases in asynchronous pacing. Magnet application will also lead to a specific pacing rate dictated by the manufacturer and model of the generator as well as its battery status (BOS, RRT, EOS).**

Connector Block or Header

The connector block is molded out of a biocompatible plastic material such as clear epoxy. This plastic connector lies on top of the pacemaker's metal case and provides the connection between the pacemaker generator and the lead(s). There are ports to accept each of the pacing leads. Single- and dual-chamber pacemakers have one and two ports, respectively, while cardiac resynchronization devices have a third port for the left ventricular lead. Depending on the manufacturer and model of the generator, there are one or two screws for each lead that must be tightened to secure the lead in the pacemaker. There is a feed-through wire that is covered by glass or sapphire that runs from each lead into the generator. The generator itself is contained in a titanium metal case, and both the case and connector block are hermetically sealed so that body fluids are kept out.

Implantable Device Codes

There is an official terminology for designating the functionality and programming of pacemaker generators that is known as the North American Society of Pacing and Electrophysiology/British Pacing and Electrophysiology Group Generic (NBG) pacemaker code. The common designation for pacemaker function consists of three letters and an optional fourth letter R (**Table 5.2**). The first of the three letters designating pacemaker function indicates

Table 5.2   Letter Code for Pacemakers

FIRST POSITION CHAMBER(S) PACED	SECOND POSITION CHAMBER(S) SENSED	THIRD POSITION RESPONSE TO SENSING	FOURTH POSITION RATE MODULATION
A=atrium	A=atrium	T=triggered	R=rate modulation
V=ventricle	V=ventricle	I=inhibited	
D=dual (A+V)	D=dual (A+V)	D=dual (triggered and inhibited)	
O=none	O=none	O=none	O=none

the cardiac chamber that is paced. This can be A for atrium, V for ventricle, D for both atrium and ventricle (dual chamber), and O for neither atrium nor ventricle. The second letter indicates the cardiac chamber that is sensed. Again, this can be A for atrium, V for ventricle, D for both atrium and ventricle, and O for neither. The third letter indicates the response to sensing. When a cardiac chamber is sensed, the electrical circuit in the pacemaker can respond by inhibiting any pacing output (I), triggering a pacing output (T), performing both operations (I + T = D), or doing neither (O). An example of triggering is when spontaneous atrial activity is sensed and a ventricular pacing output is triggered after the programmed AV delay, to restore AV synchrony in patients with AV block. The fourth position in the pacemaker code is for rate modulation. Usually, an R is used if rate response is programmed or available; otherwise, no letter in the fourth position is used.

Thus, using the NBG code, a VVI pacemaker indicates that the pacemaker produces electrical impulses to pace the ventricle (the first letter V), senses spontaneous ventricular activity (the second letter V), and responds to sensed ventricular activity by inhibiting pacing output (the letter I in VVI). A DDD pacemaker paces both the atrium and the ventricle (dual-chamber pacing, the first letter D in DDD) and senses both the atrium and the ventricle (dual-chamber sensing, the second letter D in DDD). Atrial activity can inhibit an atrial output (I response) and trigger a ventricular output (T response). The dual-response I and T is represented by the third letter D in DDD. Sensing of ventricular activity through the ventricular channel can only inhibit ventricular output.

> **The NBG code has four positions that are commonly used: chamber(s) paced, chamber(s) sensed, response to sensing, and rate modulation. A DDDR pacemaker paces the atrium and the ventricle, senses both chambers, has a dual response to sensing (inhibited and triggered), and has rate response. The complete NBG code has a fifth position for multisite pacing, but it is rarely used.**

A magnet placed over the pacemaker generator disables the sensing function of the pacemaker and by doing so makes the second letter O. Because sensing is disabled, neither inhibition nor triggering is possible, making the third letter also O. For example, a magnet placed over a pacemaker programmed VVI will make the pacemaker function in the VOO mode. A magnet placed over a DDD pacemaker will change the pacemaker function to DOO. Once the magnet is removed, the pacemaker function will return to its original setting.

Placing a magnet over a pacemaker may be done during surgery to avoid inhibition of the pacemaker by the electrical cautery often used in the operating room. Alternatively, the pacemaker can be programmed to VOO or DOO prior to the surgery and reprogrammed to the original setting after the surgery. These approaches may be necessary in a pacemaker-dependent patient, but they are not advisable and may be detrimental in a patient with a spontaneous rhythm who needs only occasional pacing.

> **A magnet placed over a pacemaker temporarily disables sensing, converting it to a VOO, AOO, or DOO mode. Using a magnet or temporarily programming an asynchronous pacing mode can be useful when there is a high risk of EMI, such as with electrocautery, in a pacemaker-dependent patient.**

Suggested Readings

Hayes DL, Wang PJ, Reynolds DW, et al. Interference with cardiac pacemakers by cellular telephones. *N Engl J Med.* 1997;336:1473–1479.

Kroll MW, Levine PA. Pacemaker and implantable cardioverter-defibrillator circuitry. In: Ellenbogen KA, Kay GN, Lau C-P, eds. *Clinical Cardiac Pacing, Defibrillation, and Resynchronization Therapy,* 3rd ed. Philadelphia: Saunders Elsevier; 2007:261–278.

Sanders RS. The pulse generator. In: Kusumoto FM, Goldschlager NF, eds. *Cardiac Pacing for the Clinician,* 2nd ed. New York: Springer; 2008:47–71.

6 ■ Implantation Techniques

Gustavo Lopera, MD, and Anne B. Curtis, MD

A permanent pacemaker system consists of a pacemaker generator and a variable number of leads. These leads are placed in specific cardiac chambers and connected to the pacemaker generator for sensing of intrinsic activity and pacing in the absence of spontaneous electrical activity.

As discussed in Chapter 1, the first successful implantation of a cardiac pacemaker occurred in 1958. The earliest pacemakers were implanted by thoracotomy. Subsequent improvements in transvenous electrodes, in use since 1958, allowed the development of transvenous implantation techniques, leading to total transvenous implantation of cardiac pacemakers by 1962. Since then, transvenous techniques have been the preferred implantation method due to lower procedural morbidity and mortality and better acceptance by patients. Nonetheless, the thoracotomy approach is still required in those instances in which the transvenous approach is not possible due to venous occlusion/stenosis, infection, and/or certain congenital or structural abnormalities.

Different transvenous and thoracotomy techniques have been described. Knowledge of these techniques will help the physician select the best technique that will suit a specific patient in any given clinical scenario.

Patient Preparation

The key to a successful procedure is adequate knowledge of the patient's medical history, performance of a physical examination, and preprocedure laboratory testing. Knowledge of the patient's medical condition will help the physician anticipate and prevent complications. For example, warfarin therapy is usually discontinued 3 to 4 days prior to an elective pacemaker implantation. Another example is that patients with severe tricuspid regurgitation may require long sheaths and active fixation leads to allow stable positioning of the right ventricular pacing lead. Requirements for preoperative evaluation are summarized in **Table 6.1**.

Logistic Requirements

Permanent pacemakers are usually implanted in a surgical environment, either the cardiac catheterization laboratory or a fluoroscopy-equipped operating room. The operator and supporting staff should be qualified individuals with special training in surgical

Table 6.1   Preoperative Requirements

PREPROCEDURE REQUIREMENTS	COMMENTS
Adequate documentation of the indication for permanent pacemaker implantation	Follow ACC/AHA/HRS guidelines.
Informed consent	Should include: indications, risks, and benefits of the procedure as well as treatment alternatives.
Detailed history and physical examination	Emphasis on aspects that could complicate or preclude performance of the implantation procedure, such as active local or systemic infection, local dermatitis, history of radiation therapy or manipulation of the central circulation, previous surgeries, and allergies.
Preprocedure laboratory testing	Complete blood count, basic metabolic panel, PT/INR, PTT, chest x-ray, and urinalysis are recommended.
	All efforts should be made to correct and treat infections and bleeding disorders that could increase the risk of preventable complications.

Table 6.1 (Continued)

Preprocedure Requirements	Comments
Anticoagulation	Heparin should be discontinued 4–6 hours and enoxaparin 8–12 hours prior to the procedure. ASA and clopidogrel are usually continued in patients with drug-eluting stents to avoid the risk of acute stent thrombosis.
Medications	Oral hypoglycemic drugs and diuretics are usually withheld, whereas the dose of insulin is halved.
Vein access	At least one upper extremity 18-gauge saline lock is necessary for administration of fluid, IV drugs, and performance of a venogram when needed.
Antibiotic prophylaxis	Patients are usually given 1 gram of IV cefazolin or vancomycin (if allergic to penicillin) 1 hour prior to the procedure.

techniques and treatment of acute cardiovascular conditions/complications. Minimal room requirements include:

1. ECG, blood pressure, and pulse oximetry monitoring
2. Biphasic external defibrillator
3. Adequate radiography/fluoroscopy and room lighting
4. Resuscitation equipment

Most procedures can be performed with local anesthesia and moderate conscious sedation with IV fentanyl and midazolam. However, a small percentage of patients (e.g., mentally challenged, demented, those with low pain tolerance) will need deep conscious sedation and/or general anesthesia.

The key to a successful pacemaker implantation is adequate knowledge of the patient's medical history and preprocedure evaluation. Emphasis should be given to factors that could increase the risk of bleeding and infection in order to minimize the risk of preventable complications.

Transvenous Techniques

Cephalic vein cut-down and percutaneous axillary and subclavian vein access are the preferred techniques for transvenous implantation of pacemaker leads. However, a small number of patients with venous thrombosis or stenosis, abandoned pacemaker leads, and infections of the upper extremity veins may require alternative transvenous approaches, such as external/internal jugular or iliofemoral vein access.

Venography

Venography can provide valuable information during pacemaker implantation procedures. It can easily be performed by injecting 10–20 cc of diluted IV-contrast media into a cubital or antecubital vein before or during the procedure (**Figure 6.1A**). The venogram helps to identify venous thrombosis and stenosis that will allow selection of an alternative pacing site before any skin incision or puncture of an upper extremity vein is attempted, thus avoiding unnecessary venous punctures and incisions or the need to switch procedural sites after the procedure has begun. It also permits a definitive demonstration of the course or trajectory of the target veins in the deltopectoral area, which varies from person to person, reducing the number of attempts for cannulation of the selected vein. Knowledge of the exact trajectory of the vein in the deltopectoral area also allows the creation of a smaller incision just on top of the known course of the vein. Venography also facilitates extrathoracic venipuncture, which decreases the risk of pneumothorax, hemothorax, and costoclavicular pacemaker lead compression (see Figure 6.1A).

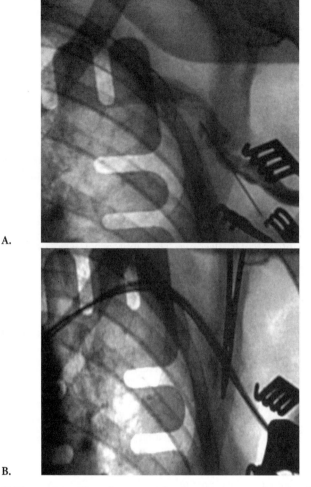

A.

B.

■ Figure 6.1   Use of venography for placement of pacing leads

A. Venogram. Demonstrates the course or trajectory of the target veins in the deltopectoral area. Defibrillation patches are observed in the background.

B. Double wire technique. One or more additional standard J-tip wires can be inserted through a sheath to allow advancement of additional introducer sheaths, avoiding the need for further vein punctures. Once the guide wires have been inserted into the first introducer sheath, the latter is removed and separate introducer sheaths are advanced over each guide wire.

> Venography allows identification of venous thrombosis/stenosis
> before a skin incision is made and facilitates puncture of
> extrathoracic veins, decreasing the risk of pneumothorax,
> hemothorax, and costoclavicular lead compression.

Cephalic Vein Cut-Down

The cephalic vein cut-down technique has certain real advantages for pacemaker implantation, because there is no risk of hemothorax or pneumothorax and minimal risk of costoclavicular lead compression. The cephalic approach is particularly useful in patients on chronic anticoagulation with aspirin and clopidogrel, because these medications sometimes cannot be discontinued before the procedure in patients with drug-eluting stents and other approaches would significantly increase the risk of hemothorax and vascular bleeding. This approach is also useful in patients with marked left ventricular dysfunction or severe emphysema who could be seriously affected by a pneumothorax, which would otherwise be well tolerated in different patient populations. Another advantage of the cephalic vein cut-down approach is minimal risk of costoclavicular lead compression. It has been reported that 93 percent of all pacemaker-lead fractures occur in the segment of the lead medial to venous entry, and costoclavicular compression has been implicated. Leads entering a vein medial to the first rib are particularly susceptible to entrapment by the subclavius muscle or the costoclavicular ligament that could result in lead fracture or insulation breaks, and this risk is highest with direct subclavian vein puncture.

Cephalic vein cut-down: technique

A skin incision is made parallel to and slightly medial to the deltopectoral groove. The skin incision is explored down to the prepectoral fascia using blunt and sharp dissection. In most patients, the cephalic vein is found in the fat tissue that separates the deltoid and pectoral muscles, but it can be absent or unusable in up to 20 percent of patients. Once the vein is dissected, proximal and distal hemostatic sutures, such as nonabsorbable 2-0 silk, are placed around it. The distal suture can be tied down before or after venotomy is attempted, whereas the proximal suture is loosely tied down over the remaining subcutaneous/vein tissue at the end of the procedure. A venotomy is performed with an 11 blade scalpel or small scissors, or alternatively an 18-gauge angiocath can be inserted into the vein. A standard J wire or flexible Glidewire (manufactured by Terumo Medical Corporation, Somerset, NJ) is advanced under fluoroscopy into the inferior vena cava (IVC). Positioning of the guide wire in the IVC confirms venous access before vascular dilation with an introducer sheath, avoiding any accidental dilatation of an arterial vessel. A tear-away SafeSheath introducer (manufactured by Pressure Products of San Pedro, California) is advanced over the guide wire under fluoroscopic guidance. This sheath combines the convenience of a tear-away introducer, to facilitate sheath removal after lead placement, with a hemostatic valve to prevent back bleeding and risk of air embolism. In most cases, a standard 13-cm sheath will allow lead placement in the desired cardiac chamber. However, patients with tortuous veins will require a 25-cm long sheath or specially designed tear-away sheaths to circumvent anomalous anatomy and allow adequate lead positioning.

Tear-away SafeSheath introducers facilitate lead advancement to the selected cardiac chamber while decreasing back bleeding and the risk of air embolization.

Double and triple wire technique

Once the introducer sheath is inserted into a central vein, one to two additional standard J-tip wires can be inserted to allow advancement of additional introducer sheaths, avoiding the need for further vein punctures and, therefore, reducing risks (**Figure 6.1B**). Two sheaths are usually required for dual-chamber pacemakers and three sheaths for biventricular pacemaker procedures. Most conventional pacemaker leads can be inserted through a 7 F introducer if the guide wire is not retained or a 9 F introducer when the guide wire is retained. This technique is applicable to any transvenous method.

While retaining the guide wire reduces the risk of additional venous access, having multiple leads in the same access site may make it more difficult to manipulate one lead into its proper location without affecting the placement of contiguous leads. For this reason, particularly with biventricular device implantation requiring three leads, combinations of access sites such as cephalic and subclavian may be used.

Cephalic vein cut-down has the lowest risk of costoclavicular lead compression and pneumothorax, but it requires more tissue dissection, which could increase the duration of the procedure.

Subclavian Approach

For many operators, the subclavian approach is the preferred route to access the central veins due to its speed, simplicity, and minimal soft-tissue dissection requirements. The main disadvantage is the higher risk of lead compression, hemothorax, and pneumothorax, especially when the subclavian vein is cannulated medial to the first rib.

Blind percutaneous technique

After application of local anesthesia, a 5 F micropuncture needle connected to a syringe is inserted at the junction of the mid and distal thirds of the clavicle. The needle is directed toward the clavicle; once the clavicle is reached, the needle is directed inferiorly just below the clavicle and advanced, aiming toward the junction of the clavicle and the first rib. Negative pressure is applied to the syringe until blood return is observed. The micropuncture wire is advanced through the needle under fluoroscopic guidance into the IVC to confirm venous access. A 5 F dilator is advanced over the

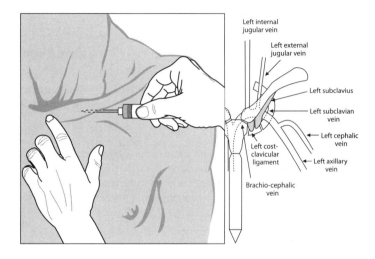

Left internal
jugular vein

Left external
jugular vein

Left subclavius

Left subclavian
vein

Left cephalic
vein

Left cost-
clavicular
ligament

Left axillary
vein

Brachio-cephalic
vein

■ **Figure 6.2   Anatomy of upper extremity veins**

For blind percutaneous access, the tip of the needle is directed under the head of the clavicle, toward the juncture of the clavicle and the first rib.

guide wire. The micropuncture guide wire is then exchanged for a standard 0.325 J wire. Alternatively, a standard access needle that accepts a 0.325 J wire can be used directly to access the subclavian vein. If there is difficulty entering the subclavian vein, the needle can be advanced under fluoroscopy. The tip of the needle will generally be seen to course directly under the head of the clavicle when access to the venous system is obtained (**Figure 6.2**).

A skin incision is then made in the infraclavicular area, parallel to and at least 2 cm below the clavicle to avoid any close contact of the leads/pulse generator with the clavicle. The skin incision is explored down to the prepectoral fascia using blunt and sharp dissection. The J wire is tunneled through the subcutaneous tissue into the pocket, if it has not been incorporated into the incision already. A tear-away SafeSheath introducer is advanced over the guide wire under fluoroscopic guidance.

Venogram-guided technique

This technique is similar to the blind percutaneous technique, except that the venogram permits direct visualization of the vein, allowing targeting of the vein lateral to the first rib. This approach theoretically can decrease the risk of lead compression, pneumothorax, hemothorax, and the number of attempts necessary before successful cannulation is achieved.

> The subclavian approach provides fast access to the central circulation and shorter procedure duration. However, it is associated with a higher risk of costoclavicular lead compression and pneumothorax.

Axillary Approach

The axillary vein is a continuation of the subclavian vein at the lateral border of the first rib. The vein runs 1–2 cm medial and parallel to the deltopectoral groove. The axillary approach offers similar advantages to the cephalic vein cut-down approach. However, its extrathoracic segment is usually deeper than the cephalic and subclavian veins, between the pectoralis major and minor. Advancement of introducer sheaths through the pectoralis major may be technically difficult, especially when the angle into the vein is greater than 60°. In these cases, introduction of a stiffer guide wire can allow advancement of the introducer sheath, avoiding the risk of vascular injuries when excessive force is applied to the introducer sheath and the standard J guide wire cannot provide adequate support.

Blind percutaneous technique

The deltopectoral groove and coracoid process are palpated. A skin incision is then made 1–2 cm medial and parallel to the deltopectoral groove. The skin incision is explored down to the prepectoral fascia using blunt and sharp dissection. A 5 F micropuncture needle or Cook needle connected to a saline syringe is advanced through the pectoralis muscle. The needle is advanced parallel to the deltopectoral groove about 1–2 cm medial at an angle of 45°. Under fluoroscopic guidance, the needle is advanced toward the first rib just under the clavicle. It is essential to observe that the tip of the needle is always over the rib to avoid the risk of pneumothorax. Once the first rib is reached, negative pressure is applied to the syringe as the needle is withdrawn slowly until blood return is observed. A guide wire and an introducer sheath are subsequently advanced into the vein as just described.

Venogram-guided technique

The technique is similar to the blind percutaneous technique, except that the venogram permits direct visualization of the vein, allowing targeting of the most lateral/extrathoracic aspects of the vein, as shown in Figure 6.1A. Again, one may decrease the risk of pneumothorax, hemothorax, and the number of attempts before successful cannulation is achieved.

External and Internal Jugular Approach

Although widely used in the early years of transvenous implantation of permanent pacemakers, the jugular vein approach is currently reserved for patients in whom the axillary, subclavian, or cephalic veins cannot be used. Of note, the phrenic and vagus nerves lie posterior to the internal jugular vein, and injury to these nerves has been reported with this technique.

Iliofemoral Approach

When transvenous implantation of pacemakers via the upper extremity veins is not possible, patients are usually referred for thoracotomy and epicardial lead placement. However, the iliofemoral approach offers a less-invasive option with low complication rates. The incidence of atrial lead dislodgement is relatively high with this method. Reported cases of thrombophlebitis and infections are relatively low, but still higher than for deltopectoral implants.

Thoracotomy Techniques

Thoracotomy techniques are reserved for patients in whom the transvenous route is not possible, such as in patients with venous thrombosis/stenosis, high risk of recurrent bacteremia, intracavitary shunts with a high risk of thromboembolic events, and previous cardiac surgery that prevents transvenous pacing, such as tricuspid valve replacement.

Thoracotomy techniques can be performed via sternotomy or thoracotomy. In recent years, less-invasive mini-thoracotomy techniques have been introduced. In particular, the transatrial mini-thoracotomy technique seems to offer some advantages over other thoracotomy techniques, since conventional leads can be inserted into the right atrium and ventricle via the right atrium. Insertion of leads for pacing the left ventricle through the CS has also been described with this technique.

Thoracotomy and nonconventional transvenous techniques may be used in patients in need of pacing therapy but with contraindications or inaccessibility to traditional transvenous methods.

Creation of the Pacemaker Pocket

The pacemaker pocket is usually created in the plane of the prepectoral fascia deep to the subcutaneous fatty tissue. It is important to create an even plane to avoid inappropriate motion of the pulse generator in the pocket, which can lead to excessive pressure on the skin that could cause pain and/or erosion of the pacemaker. The pocket should also be sufficiently medial to avoid the axilla and inferior to the clavicle in order to avoid interference with the patient's shoulder motion.

Technique

The skin incision is explored down to the prepectoral fascia using blunt and sharp dissection. Manual dissection, electrocautery, and/or blunt dissection with blunt tip Metzenbaum scissors may be used to create a pocket in the prepectoral fascia. The size of the pocket should be enough to accommodate the pulse generator and leads. Small pockets can cause pain and/or erosion of the pacemaker pocket and large pockets can cause excessive motion of the generator in the pocket.

Emaciated patients and individuals with thin dermal layers and little subcutaneous tissue or scars in the infraclavicular region may benefit from subpectoral pockets to accommodate the leads and pulse generator in the space between the pectoralis major and minor.

Small pacemaker pockets can cause pain and/or erosion of the pacemaker pocket and large pockets can cause excessive motion of the generator in the pocket.

Lead Placement

Positioning of pacing leads is similar for passive and active fixation leads. Passive fixation leads require adequate anchorage of the lead tines into the trabeculated endocardial surface to achieve a stable lead position, whereas active fixation leads only require deployment of a retractable or nonretractable screw at the tip.

Right Atrium

Insertion of a pacing lead into the RAA remains the preferred site for atrial lead placement, because it offers significant stability for chronic pacing and simple anatomic landmarks during implantation. In brief, the lead is advanced through the introducer sheath into the lower right atrium with a straight stylet. In the case of most active fixation atrial leads, the stylet is then exchanged for a preformed J-tipped stylet, and the lead is slowly pulled back as the J-tipped stylet is introduced. Slight counter- and clockwise rotation is applied to the J-tipped stylet to allow positioning into the RAA. In most patients, a slight jump is appreciated when the lead tip enters the RAA. On fluoroscopy, a typical to-and-fro horizontal motion of the lead tip is appreciated as the appendage exhibits more vigorous contractions when compared to other segments of the right atrium. Oblique radiographic projections will help in the correct identification of the RAA; the lead tip will point anterior in the right anterior oblique (RAO) fluoroscopy projection and toward the left in the left anterior oblique (LAO) fluoroscopy projection. The LAO projection also helps to identify the lateral wall of the atrium, which should be avoided due to a higher risk of perforation and lead dislodgement. When the lead is placed in a satisfactory position in the RAA, the screw is advanced into the atrial tissue and the stylet is pulled back in a quick, smooth motion to minimize the chance of lead dislodgement.

Passive fixation atrial leads have tines at the tip to stabilize them in the RAA. Such leads have a preformed J shape. The lead is advanced into the heart using a straight stylet. As the stylet is pulled back, the J shape is restored and the lead is positioned in the RAA.

A properly placed right atrial lead will have a J shape on fluoroscopy, and the J will not open beyond about 80° on full inspiration. Leaving either too little or too much slack in a passive fixation atrial lead will increase the chances of dislodgement. An active fixation lead that is placed well in the heart can accept more slack.

The interatrial septum or Bachmann's bundle pacing, multisite right atrial pacing, and biatrial pacing have been proposed as alternative pacing sites with theoretical advantages in terms of interatrial conduction and prevention of atrial tachyarrhythmias. However, to date there have been no consistent data from randomized trials to support the use of alternative site pacing in preference to RAA pacing, and the latter has the advantage of simplicity and excellent lead stability.

Right Ventricle

Insertion of a pacing lead into the RVA remains the most frequently used pacing site, because it offers great stability for chronic pacing. In brief, the lead is advanced through an introducer sheath into the right atrium with a straight stylet. This stylet is then exchanged for a stylet that is curved by the operator to allow advancement of the lead into the right ventricle across the tricuspid valve. Once in the right ventricle, the lead can be further advanced into the right ventricular outflow tract. This maneuver is encouraged in order to be certain that the lead is in the right ventricle itself and not the CS or middle cardiac vein. The curved stylet is then exchanged for a straight stylet, which is advanced into the lead body as the lead is gradually pulled back from the right ventricular outflow tract. Once free in the right ventricle, the lead is advanced to the RVA or right ventricular septum under fluoroscopic guidance. A soft straight stylet is recommended to avoid transmission of excessive force to the lead tip that could cause perforation of the right ventricle. Additionally, the straight stylet can be pulled back a few millimeters from the lead tip to allow greater flexibility of the tip as the lead is introduced further into the right ventricle, decreasing the risk of cardiac perforation. For placement in the right ventricular septum, an active fixation lead is essential. Either an active or a passive fixation lead may be used in the RVA.

Pressure-mapping technique

Slight pressure is applied to the lead tip until contact with the myocardium is achieved. Under fluoroscopy, the lead tip will move with the ventricle with each cardiac contraction. Subsequently, the external analyzer cables are connected to the lead electrodes to verify adequate sensing before the lead is screwed into the myocardium, in the case of active fixation leads. This technique will avoid fixing the lead in suboptimal sites, decreasing the number of times the lead is screwed and unscrewed in the right ventricle, and also decreasing the risk of cardiac perforation. Another problem that can develop when the screw is fixed and unfixed multiple times is entrapment of tissue in the screw. This tissue can prevent adequate fixation of the lead in new sites and ultimately render the lead unusable.

This mapping technique can also be used for selection of the atrial pacing site. In general, a sensed R wave greater than 5 mV in the right ventricle and a sensed P wave greater than 1.5 mV in the right atrium are considered acceptable before the lead is screwed into the myocardium.

> **Measurement of the sensed P or R wave before screwing an active fixation lead into the myocardium can easily be performed, decreasing the number of times the lead is screwed and unscrewed and, hence, decreasing the risk of cardiac perforation and tissue entrapment in the screw.**

Adjusting lead slack

Once the lead is positioned in the desired location in the right ventricle, the straight stylet is pulled back into the right atrium or superior vena cava (SVC) and the position of the lead body is adjusted until adequate slack is observed on fluoroscopy. Excessive lead slack can cause undue pressure on the distal lead tip, which can cause migration of the lead into the pericardial space (late perforation). Inadequate slack is associated with higher rates of lead dislodgement.

Introducer sheaths

Introducer sheaths are removed either as soon as the lead is advanced into the heart, or they may be removed after positioning of the lead, in the case of difficult access or difficult maneuverability of the lead in the heart.

Patients with tortuous veins, dilated cardiac chambers, rotated cardiac chambers, acquired or congenital cardiac anomalies, and valvular abnormalities may require special tear-away introducer sheaths. For example, patients with tortuous veins may require long 25 cm introducer sheaths. Patients with severe tricuspid regurgitation or restrictive cardiomyopathy may require introduction of a multipurpose tear-away sheath into the right ventricle for direct lead delivery, which can be achieved by advancing the multipurpose sheath over a 6 F Josephson or any other deflectable tip catheter.

Alternative right ventricular pacing sites

Pacing of the right ventricular outflow tract is a safe and effective alternative to right ventricular apical and right ventricular septal pacing. Acute hemodynamics appear to be superior with right ventricular outflow tract pacing compared to right ventricular apical pacing. However, similar results have not consistently been shown with chronic pacing studies, possibly because the length of follow-up has not been sufficiently long. In multiple clinical trials, cumulative right ventricular pacing greater than 40 percent of the time has been associated with a higher risk of AF and heart failure. Ongoing clinical trials are investigating whether using alternative sites or biventricular pacing rather than right ventricular apical pacing will avoid these problems.

Pacing of the right ventricular septum is usually associated with a narrower QRS compared to right ventricular apical pacing and has a lower risk of perforation. This is especially important in patients with a thin and dilated right ventricular chamber.

> **Right ventricular septal and right ventricular apical positions remained the most frequently used sites for right ventricular pacing. Right ventricular septal pacing is associated with a lower rate of cardiac perforation than right ventricular apical pacing.**

Left Ventricle

CRT has emerged as a highly effective therapy for patients with advanced heart failure. Results from observational studies and randomized clinical trials of CRT have consistently demonstrated significant improvements in quality of life, functional status, exercise capacity, and survival in patients with NYHA class III and IV heart failure symptoms, LVEF ≤ 35 percent and ventricular dyssynchrony. The latter is defined in current guidelines by a QRS duration ≥120 msec, typically with a LBBB or intraventricular conduction delay. CRT is accomplished with biventricular pacing, in which one pacing lead is placed in the right ventricle and another lead in the left ventricle via the CS. The great majority of the patients who receive CRT are in sinus rhythm, and therefore a third lead is placed in the right atrium for atrial-synchronous biventricular pacing.

Clinical trials of CRT have consistently demonstrated significant improvements in quality of life, functional status, exercise capacity, and survival in patients with severe systolic heart failure and ECG evidence of ventricular dyssynchrony.

Technique

Separate venous access for the left ventricular lead to avoid excessive friction with the atrial and right ventricular leads is recommended, but it is not a requirement. A 9 Fr tear-away SafeSheath introducer is advanced over the guide wire under fluoroscopic guidance. Transvenous placement of the left ventricular epicardial lead requires cannulation of the CS for performance of a selective CS venogram and delivery of the left ventricular pacing lead.

Sheath selection

Multiple tear-away and split-away delivery sheaths are widely available. Different preformed shapes are available to facilitate CS cannulation according to the patient's anatomy, such as severe right atrial enlargement and inferior or superior displacement of the CS os. As a general rule, the size of the secondary or proximal curve of the sheath/outer catheter should match the horizontal diameter of the right atrium. Thus, the larger the right atrium, the larger the secondary or proximal curve on the sheath/outer catheter should be. Selection of the primary or distal curve depends on the inferior, neutral, or superior displacement of the CS os. For example, left Amplatz-type sheaths/outer catheters exhibit a superiorly directed primary curve and are very helpful in cannulation of a superiorly displaced CS os. Multipurpose A2 catheters have a tip that can be directed inferiorly or superiorly when advanced through an outer catheter/sheath (angiographic or inner/outer catheter technique) (**Figure 6.3**).

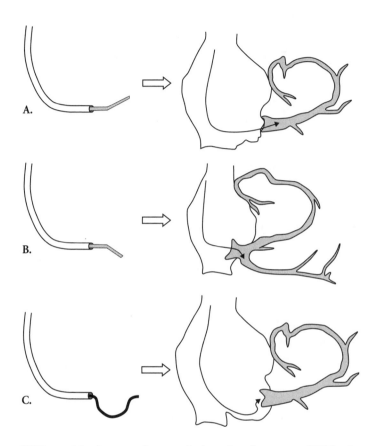

■ **Figure 6.3   Inner catheter technique for placement of CS leads**

Cannulation of the CS can be facilitated with the use of inner catheters in the case of an inferiorly or superiorly displaced CS ostium.

Adapted with permission from Singh JP, Houser S, Heist EK, Ruskin JN. The Coronary Venous Anatomy: A Segmental Approach to Aid Cardiac Resynchronization Therapy. *Journal of the American College of Cardiology*. 2005;46:68–74.

Coronary sinus cannulation

Successful cannulation of the CS requires an understanding of the anatomic changes in the remodeled heart. In most cases, upward shift of the long axis and counter-clockwise rotation of the short

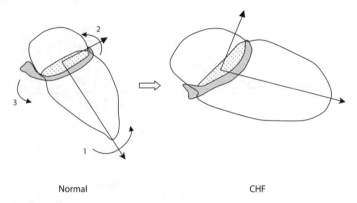

Normal   CHF

■ Figure 6.4   Effects of cardiac remodeling in heart failure

Cardiac remodeling causes displacement of the CS os.

Adapted with permission from Singh JP, Houser S, Heist EK, Ruskin JN. The Coronary Venous Anatomy: A Segmental Approach to Aid Cardiac Resynchronization Therapy. *Journal of the American College of Cardiology*. 2005;46:68–74.

axis of the heart moves the CS to a relatively lower and posterior position (**Figure 6.4**). The selected sheath for cannulation of the CS is usually advanced through a 9 F introducer sheath.

Several techniques for CS cannulation have been described:

1. Electrophysiologic technique

    A 6 F Josephson, 6 F CSL catheter, or any deflectable tip catheter is advanced to the right atrium and used to cannulate the CS. In brief, the catheter is advanced to the floor of the right atrium. Once at this level, counter-clockwise rotation is applied as the catheter is advanced under fluoroscopic guidance. Recording of EGMs will help to indicate when the catheter has been advanced beyond the right atrium and CS and into the right ventricle (ventricular EGMs with no atrial EGMs on the distal poles of the catheter). In the LAO projection, the catheter is advanced aiming toward the spine. CS cannulation may be verified by identification of the typical CS EGM, which has dual deflections (atrial and ventricular signals). Once the CS is cannulated, the sheath is advanced over the electrode catheter.

2. Angiographic or outer/inner catheter technique
   A coronary angiographic catheter (JR, AL, or multipurpose) is advanced over the guide wire into the right ventricle under fluoroscopic guidance. Once in the right ventricle, the catheter and guide wire are gradually pulled back into the right atrium as gentle counter-clockwise rotation is applied. The wire is advanced under fluoroscopy, aiming toward the spine in the LAO projection until the CS is cannulated. The angiographic catheter is advanced over the wire into the CS and the selected sheath is advanced over this catheter. A variation on this technique is to use the outer sheath alone, advance it to the right ventricle, and then direct it toward the CS as it is pulled back with counter-clockwise rotation (**Figure 6.5**).

3. Sheathless technique
   Direct cannulation of the CS is attempted using only a lead stylet or wire manipulation. Lead delivery is performed without the CS sheath and CS venogram. When successful, this technique is faster and could decrease the complications associated with CS sheaths, such as CS dissection or lead dislodgement.

Access to the CS may be accomplished with electrode catheters and intracardiac EGM monitoring, angiographic catheters with contrast injections, or by direct advancement of guide wires.

CS venography, branch selection, and left ventricular lead delivery

CS venography allows the identification of the optimal CS branches for pacing. It also permits lead selection, based on the size of the target CS branch. For example, straight bipolar or unipolar leads are used for smaller branches whereas bipolar leads with preformed curves are used for large veins.

A venogram can be performed by injecting a small amount of contrast directly into the sheath or through a balloon-tipped catheter (occlusive technique). Some cases might require both techniques for adequate identification of CS branches (**Figure 6.6**).

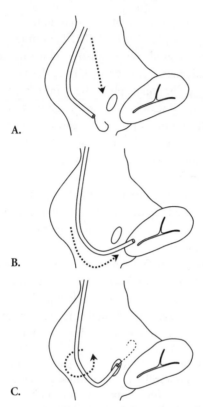

■ Figure 6.5 Angiographic technique for CS lead placement

The catheter is advanced into the right ventricle and then directed toward the CS as it is pulled back with counter-clockwise rotation.

Adapted with permission from Singh JP, Houser S, Heist EK, Ruskin JN. The Coronary Venous Anatomy: A Segmental Approach to Aid Cardiac Resynchronization Therapy. *Journal of the American College of Cardiology.* 2005;46:68–74.

Several multicenter studies have confirmed that the left ventricular lead should be placed in a posterior or lateral vein, or, as a last resort, into an anterolateral CS branch. On the contrary, stimulation of the anterior wall or apex via the middle and great cardiac veins has little to no advantage and could even have adverse hemodynamic effects.

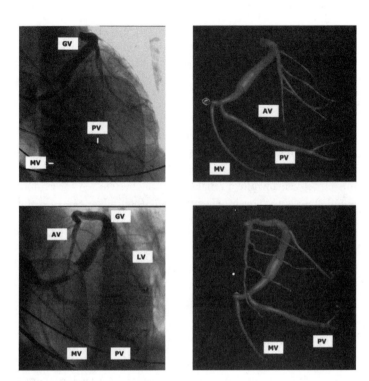

■ Figure 6.6   CS venograms

The posterior and lateral branches are the preferred sites for pacing. MV=
middle cardiac vein; PV= posterior vein; LV= lateral vein; GV= great cardiac vein; AV= anterior cardiac vein.

Used with permission from Singh JP, Houser S, Heist EK, Ruskin JN. The Coronary
Venous Anatomy: A Segmental Approach to Aid Cardiac Resynchronization Therapy. *Journal of the American College of Cardiology.* 2005;46:68–74.

Lead delivery to desired anatomic locations is limited by lead
design and variations in CS anatomy, such as acutely angled or tortuous CS branches. Initially, left ventricle leads could only be delivered via stylet-driven manipulation of the tip. Subsequently, OTW
leads were developed, allowing lead delivery to sites not accessible
with stylet-driven leads. Although OTW leads allow targeting of
multiple CS branches, delivery failure can still be observed in some

cases. Most of these failures are due to inadequate lead support during delivery. In recent years, telescopic techniques have allowed the delivery of left ventricular pacing leads to sites requiring additional lead support, such as acutely angled or tortuous CS branches.

Telescopic techniques are a variation of the outer/inner catheter technique. Once the outer catheter is in the main CS, an inner catheter with a preselected tip shape is advanced over an angioplasty wire. A hockey stick inner catheter may be useful for tortuous target veins, while a renal curve may be selected for acutely angulated veins. The inner catheter is then advanced into the selected branch over the angioplasty wire and the lead is delivered through the inner catheter.

The left ventricular lead for resynchronization therapy should preferentially be placed in a posterior or lateral branch of the CS to achieve good outcomes.

Electronic repositioning

High left ventricular pacing thresholds and phrenic nerve stimulation are frequent problems during left ventricular lead implantation. Previously, the only solution to this problem was to use a more proximal segment of the same branch or to use a different branch. However, proximal segments are less stable and associated with higher dislodgement rates, and not all patients have more than one optimal lateral or posterior branch suitable for pacing. Newer devices allow programming of different configurations for left ventricular pacing, such as tip-to-ring, ring-to-tip, tip-to-coil (for an ICD lead), ring-to-coil, and so forth. Different electronic configurations can be tested at implantation, often times allowing left ventricular pacing in adequate/desirable anatomical positions that have less-than-acceptable pacing thresholds or phrenic nerve stimulation with standard pacing configurations.

Intraoperative Measurements

Optimal placement of pacemaker leads involves not only the selection of an adequate and stable anatomic site for pacing but also entails the selection of a pacing site with satisfactory electrophysiologic properties to support chronic pacing in the selected cardiac chamber. The latter can be accomplished by the determination of the pacing and sensing thresholds as well as lead impedances at the time of the procedure and before closure of the pacemaker pocket. An external pacing system analyzer is used to assess these parameters at the selected site. In brief, external cables connect the analyzer to the distal electrode of the pacing lead and the skin (unipolar) or the distal and proximal electrodes of the pacing lead (bipolar) to measure intracardiac EGMs.

The EGM has three basic components:

1. The intrinsic deflection, a rapid biphasic deflection that occurs as the myocardium adjacent to the electrode depolarizes. It is the component of the EGM that is measured or sensed, usually expressed in mV. It also exhibits the highest slew rate of the EGM. The slew rate is the rate of change of the voltage developed by the EGM and is described in volts per second.
2. Far-field potentials arise from electrical activity distant from the electrode, such as an adjacent cardiac chamber. Skeletal muscle potentials and external EMI may also produce extraneous signals that may create sensing problems.
3. The "current of injury" appears as an elevation immediately following the intrinsic deflection. Believed to be due to a small area of damaged endocardium caused by irritation from the pacemaker electrode, it lessens as time passes and is rarely seen in the chronic EGM.

The optimal sensed atrial and ventricular EGMs at the time of implantation, to secure adequate long-term sensing, should be greater than 1.5 mV and 5 mV, respectively. Less–than-optimal ventricular sensing (<5 mV) can be accepted if a slew rate >1.5 mV/ms is found.

Acceptable acute pacing thresholds should be less than 1.5 V at a 0.5-msec pulse width duration for both atrial and ventricular leads. However, higher pacing thresholds are usually accepted for leads in the left ventricle.

Lead impedances usually range from 300 to 1500 ohms, depending on the lead type.

> **Adequate sites for pacing should demonstrate P waves >1.5 mV, R waves >5 mV (sensing thresholds), and pacing thresholds <1.5 V at a 0.5-msec pulse width.**

Wound Closure and Postoperative Care

Once hemostasis has been achieved, the lead slack has been adjusted, and intraoperative testing has been found to be adequate, the leads are anchored to the pectoral fascia using nonabsorbable sutures (e.g., 2-0 Ethibon or silk) over a rubber sleeve provided with the lead. It is important to tie the sutures over the sleeve and not directly on the lead, because the latter could lead to insulation breaks and lead fractures. The pocket is then flushed with an antibiotic solution (e.g., 1 gram of cefazolin or vancomycin diluted in 0.9 percent saline). Subsequently, the selected pacemaker is attached to the leads, usually by means of screws in the header of the generator, and inserted into the pocket. Adequate connection of the leads to the pacemaker header is essential to avoid loose set screw problems that mimic lead fractures (high impedances, high pacing thresholds, and failure to capture). Slight tugging on the lead after it is screwed into the header is recommended to verify adequate connection to the header. It is important to be sure that the leads are placed deep to the generator in the pocket and without kinking or strain. Such care will minimize future lead problems and also make subsequent generator changes easier to accomplish.

The skin incision is then closed using absorbable sutures (2-0 or 3-0 Vicryl for deep layers and 4-0 for the subcuticular layer), and sterile steri-strips and a dressing are applied over the wound. The sterile dressing is usually kept on for 24 to 72 hours, whereas the steri-strips are left over the wound and are allowed to peel off spontaneously.

Adequate implantation technique mandates that there be satisfactory hemostasis. This should be confirmed after suturing the leads on the pectoral fascia over the rubber sleeves and before the pacemaker is connected to the leads.

Pulse Generator Changes

The power source in modern pacemakers is a chemical battery—lithium-iodine, in most cases. The battery voltage is dependent on the chemistry of the cell. For example, the lithium-iodine cell generates approximately 2.8 V at the beginning of its life. The longevity of a pulse generator will depend on the characteristics of the battery, the current drain of the IC, the amplitude and duration of the output impulses, frequency of stimulation, and lead impedance.

Replacement of a pulse generator is recommended within a period of weeks to months once the RRT is identified during routine pacemaker follow-up. EOL indicators denote gross pacemaker malfunction or lack of function and usually require immediate pulse generator change.

The main risk of a pulse generator change is infection of the pacemaker pocket. When compared to new implants, pulse generator changes are associated with a two- to fourfold increase in the risk of infection. Removal of the pacemaker capsule (avascular tissue) at the time of generator replacement may promote healing and possibly decrease the risk of infection.

Knowledge of a patient's underlying rhythm is essential to determine whether a temporary pacemaker may be needed during the pulse generator change. Transvenous pacemakers for backup pacing are recommended in pacemaker-dependent patients with very low (<40 bpm) or absent escape rhythms. An experienced operator may be able to remove the lead from the generator quickly and pace in a unipolar manner until the new generator is attached to the lead, thus avoiding temporary pacing. Patients with underlying heart rates greater than 40 bpm usually do not require backup transvenous pacing.

Preprocedure venograms are recommended for patients in whom a pacemaker upgrade or lead replacement is anticipated or planned.

Intraoperative testing, incision closure, and wound care are performed in a similar fashion as previously described for new implantation procedures.

Knowledge of a patient's underlying rhythm is essential during the pulse generator change. Transvenous pacemakers are recommended in pacemaker-dependent patients with very low (<40 bpm) or absent escape rhythms.

Suggested Readings

Belott PH. Blind axillary venous access. *Pacing Clin Electrophysiol.* 1999; 22:1085–1089.

Gras D, Leon AR, Fisher WG, eds. *The Road to Successful CRT Implantation: A Step-by-Step Approach*, 1st ed. Malden, MA: Blackwell Futura; 2004.

Hayes DL, Lloyd MA, Friedman PA. *Cardiac Pacing and Defibrillation: A Clinical Approach.* Armonk, NY: Futura Publishing Company; 2000.

7 ■ Basic Programming

ROBERT J. HARIMAN, MD, AND ANNE B. CURTIS, MD

Certain fundamental parameters must be programmed in any permanent pacemaker in order to get the most basic functionality. At the time of implantation, pacemaker generators are provided with nominal settings that will provide adequate pacing for most patients. However, it is essential to know what these programmed parameters are, what their purpose is, and how they should be adjusted for individual patients so they get the most benefit from their pacemakers.

Output

A pacemaker impulse consists of an electrical signal that has a certain duration (pulse width) and amplitude (voltage). Because the most essential function of a pacemaker is to provide pacing outputs to a patient with an inadequate intrinsic rhythm, one of the goals in pacemaker programming is to program the pacemaker to produce atrial and/or ventricular outputs that reliably cause atrial or ventricular depolarizations (atrial or ventricular capture). In addition to obtaining good contact during lead implantation, this goal can be achieved by programming an output with an adequately large voltage and pulse width. The implantable pacemakers available in the market today are constant voltage generators with programmable voltage outputs. Current output follows voltage changes according to Ohm's law. In addition, the pacemaker pulse width can be programmed independently from the voltage output.

In order to program the voltage output of a pacemaker, one has to determine the voltage threshold (the lowest voltage that produces a reliable atrial or ventricular depolarization at a given pulse width). The pacing threshold is determined by pacing at a high output initially and then decrementing the voltage until loss of capture is seen. The decrement in output is usually done automatically through the pacemaker programmer or pacing system analyzer, but it can also be done manually. Once the threshold is determined, the pacemaker is programmed at a higher output to provide a safety margin so that depolarization of the cardiac chamber will be accomplished reliably. As an example, a pacemaker is found to capture the ventricle at 1 V at a pulse width of 0.5 msec, while loss of capture is seen at 0.9 V and 0.5 msec. The ventricular pacing threshold is thus 1 V at a pulse width of 0.5 msec. The pacemaker might then be programmed to generate an output of 2.5 V at a 0.5 msec pulse duration. This voltage output is 2.5 times the voltage threshold. Output amplitudes that are two to three times the threshold are considered safe in causing capture reliably. With chronic pacing thresholds of about 1 V, a typical programmed output would be 2.0–3.0 V (**Table 7.1**).

It is essential to program a safe but not excessive pacing voltage, because pacing outputs that greatly exceed the pacing threshold will result in premature battery depletion. Calculation of the energy expended for different voltage outputs will help to illustrate this point. The equations used in these calculations are shown in **Table 7.2**. As shown in **Table 7.3**, the effect of doubling the voltage output is to quadruple the energy expended.

By keeping the voltage output within two to three times the voltage threshold, one minimizes the amount of energy per ventricular stimulation and maximizes the life expectancy of the pacemaker battery.

Strength-Duration Curves

Strength duration curves plot the voltage threshold (in volts) on the y-axis versus the pulse width (in msec) on the x-axis. These curves can usually be drawn automatically using a pacemaker programmer through a two-step process. First, the voltage threshold is determined at a fixed pulse width, and then the pulse width is decremented at a fixed voltage output until loss of capture is observed.

Table 7.1 Basic Programmed Parameters in Permanent Pacemakers

PARAMETER	TYPICAL VALUES
Lower rate	50–70 beats/min
Upper rate	120–150 beats/min
Pacing amplitude	2.0–3.0 V (range 1.0–7.5 V)
Pulse width	0.5 msec
Sensitivity	Ventricle, 2.0–2.8 mV Atrium, 0.5–1.0 mV
AV delay	120–300 msec (paced AV delays usually exceed sensed AV delays by about 30 msec)
Refractory periods	Ventricle, 200–250 msec Total atrial refractory period (TARP), 350–500 msec
Post ventricular atrial refractory period (PVARP)	225–400 msec

Table 7.2 Equations Used in Permanent Pacemakers

Ohm's Law: $V = I \times R$

Energy: $E = V \times I \times PD$

E=energy (microjoules, mJ); I=current (milliamperes, mA); PD=pulse duration (milliseconds, msec); R=resistance (or impedance, in ohms, Ω); V=voltage

As a rule of thumb, it is desirable to keep the pulse duration at values less than 1 msec. The reason for this is shown in **Figure 7.1**, which depicts a strength-duration curve. Thus, point A represents the ventricular pacing threshold at 1 V and 0.5 msec. As can be noted in Figure 7.1, at pulse widths approaching and beyond 1 msec, the strength-duration curve is flat. Thus, by increasing the pulse to 1.2 msec (from point A to C), the voltage

Table 7.3   Effect of a Change in Voltage on the Energy Output in a Permanent Pacemaker

Voltage = 2.5 V	Voltage = 5.0 V
Impedance = 500 Ω	Impedance = 500 Ω
I = V/R = 2.5 V/500 Ω = 5 mA	I = V/R = 5.0 V/500 Ω = 10 mA
E = 2.5 V × 5 mA × 0.5 msec = 6.25 mJ	E = 5.0 V × 10 mA × 0.5 msec = 25 mJ

threshold declines very little, and, as a result, point C is not far above the curve. This increase in pulse width significantly increases energy expenditure per stimulating pulse, and yet it does not ensure a significantly more reliable capture. Instead, by increasing the voltage from 1.0 to 2.5 V (from point A to B), point B is moved far above the curve. This example shows why one rarely uses pulse widths above 1.0 msec in pacemaker programming.

As a rule of thumb, it is desirable to keep the pulse duration for pacing at values less than 1 msec.

Pacemakers can be programmed to unipolar or bipolar pacing, provided that a bipolar pacing lead is in place. In a unipolar system, current flow is between the tip of the pacemaker lead (cathode) and the pacemaker pulse generator (anode). In a bipolar system, the anode is a proximal ring on the lead located 1 to 2 cm from the tip of the pacemaker lead, where the distal electrode is located (cathode). The current flow is then between the distal electrode and the proximal ring. The threshold can be better with either bipolar or unipolar pacing. In order to conserve the pacemaker battery, the system with the better pacing threshold may be chosen if there is a significant difference between the two. However, if the pacemaker generator is implanted adjacent to the pectoral muscle (as in a sub-pectoral implantation), it is best to avoid unipolar pacing, because this configuration can cause pectoral muscle stimulation by the current exiting from the generator can.

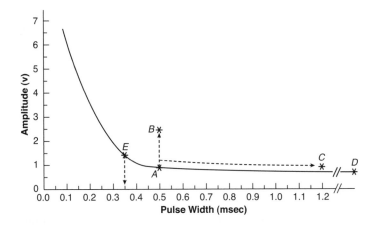

■ **Figure 7.1 Strength-duration curve**

Plotted are the pacing thresholds with pulse width (in msec) on the x-axis and amplitude (in volts) on the y-axis. See explanations for points A, B, and C in the text. Point D represents rheobase, defined as the voltage threshold at an infinitely long pulse width. Point E represents a point in the curve at a voltage amplitude twice that of point D. The pulse width for point E is termed chronaxie, which can be defined as the pulse width of a point in the strength-duration curve where the amplitude is twice the rheobase.

Sensitivity

Sensing of activity of a cardiac chamber is achieved by the pacemaker monitoring cardiac EGMs. Better contact of the pacemaker lead in the chamber of interest will lead to a larger amplitude EGM. However, sometimes areas of the heart with good contact still do not have adequate amplitude signals for sensing, such as in an area of a previous myocardial infarction. In such cases, positioning the lead in a different location will usually improve the amplitude of the sensed signal. The direction of impulse propagation will also affect EGM amplitude, but the latter is in general not predictable during routine placement of a pacemaker lead in the heart. Depending on the position of the lead and the relative sizes of different EGMs, far-field potentials from the chamber that is not intended to be sensed can be detected. The most common example of this problem is sensing of ventricular activity on the atrial lead, because of the larger ventricular muscle mass. In addition, other signals (such as the T wave or delayed activation of the ventricle associated with an intraventricular conduction delay) can be sensed inappropriately. For the ventricle, the most common way to avoid these extra signals is by programming an extended ventricular refractory period (see discussion later) or by decreasing sensitivity so that only larger signals above a certain amplitude are selectively recognized. Frequently, the latter is made possible by the large amplitude of the cardiac EGMs in the chamber of interest (P waves in the atrium and R waves in the ventricle).

At the time of pacemaker implantation, the acceptable minimum value for R waves is 5.0 mV, with values as high as 20 mV or more seen in some patients. In order to detect such signals chronically, sensitivity on the ventricular channel is usually set to 2.0–2.8 mV (see Table 7.1). P waves are generally much smaller. Ideally, they should be >2.0 mV at the time of implantation, but it may be necessary in some patients to accept values of 1.0–1.5 mV. Thus, P wave sensitivity is usually programmed to approximately 0.5 mV. Large intrinsic P or R waves or problems with far-field sensing may make it advisable to program less-sensitive settings in some patients. A key concept is that the sensitivity setting is the *minimum* signal amplitude that will be detected by the pacemaker. Thus, if one wants to program the pacemaker to be *less* sensitive, the value of the sensitivity setting is *increased*.

The polarity of sensing, unipolar or bipolar, may be programmed independently from the polarity of pacing. The larger interelectrode distance in a unipolar system (from the can to the lead tip, compared to the distal electrode to the proximal ring in a bipolar system) may result in a larger EGM. However, bipolar sensing in general provides a better slew rate (i.e., a larger rate of change, or dV/dt, of the EGM), which improves sensing. Bipolar sensing is also less prone to interference from sources such as muscle potentials, EMI, and T waves.

> The sensitivity setting is the *minimum* signal amplitude that will be detected by the pacemaker. Thus, if one wants to program the pacemaker to be *less* sensitive, the value of the sensitivity setting is *increased*.

Lower and Upper Pacing Rates

The lower pacing rate (also called lower rate limit [LRL]) in single-chamber pacing (AAI, VVI, AAIR, or VVIR) is the lowest rate of the pacemaker electrical impulses. The lower pacing rate is programmable. In a patient with a VVI pacemaker programmed to a rate of 60 beats per minute, the pacemaker output will be inhibited by ventricular activity occurring at intervals shorter than 1 second (equivalent to a heart rate faster than 60 beats per minute). In the VVI mode, the LRL is equal to the pacing rate. There is only a lower pacing rate in single-chamber pacemakers without rate-responsive programming; higher heart rates come from the patient's intrinsic cardiac activity.

In the VVIR mode, a patient with an LRL of 60 beats per minute will also have a minimum heart rate of 60 beats per minute, when the rate response sensor is not activated. However, when the rate response sensor is activated, the pacing rate will be higher than 60 beats per minute. The pacemaker will only be inhibited by intrinsic heart rates exceeding the rate dictated by the activated rate response sensor. The maximum pacing rate (also called upper rate limit [URL]) in a single-chamber rate responsive pacemaker, either AAIR or VVIR, is equal to the maximum rate of the rate response function.

In dual-chamber pacing (DDD, DDI, DDDR, and DDIR), the LRL for the atrium will determine the atrial pacing rate when the intrinsic atrial rate is slower than the programmed LRL.

Ventricular pacing then will occur only if there is no ventricular activity seen within the programmed pacemaker AV interval (also called AV delay). The programmed URL will be the ceiling for both the atrial pacing rate and the ventricular pacing rate, provided that the TARP has not been exceeded (see the discussion later). Similarly, when a pacemaker is programmed to VDD or VDDR pacing, the ceiling rate for ventricular pacing remains the URL, which in many instances may be lower than the intrinsic sinus rate. The lower rate of the URL with respect to the sinus rate may reduce the ability of ventricular pacing to track sinus rhythm in a 1:1 fashion (see the discussion on upper rate responses).

It should be noted that it is possible to program two separate URLs in DDDR pacemakers. One is the maximum tracking rate, or the maximum ventricular pacing rate based on sensed P waves. It may be set to a value lower than the maximum sensor rate to avoid rapid pacing rates during atrial tachyarrhythmias. However, lower maximum tracking rates also compromise AV synchrony during sinus tachycardia. The second URL is the maximum sensor rate, or the pacing rate determined by the programming of the rate response sensor. The actual heart rate seen in an individual patient depends solely on which heart rate is higher—the patient's intrinsic heart rate (which could exceed all programmed parameters, such as when the patient goes into AF), the tracking rate, or the sensor-driven rate.

The maximum tracking rate and the maximum sensor rate are independently programmable in DDDR pacemakers.

AV Delay

The AV delay is a programmable function in dual-chamber pacemakers. It is the interval between an atrial event (paced or spontaneous) and the paced ventricular event. The interval from a spontaneous atrial event to a ventricular pacing spike (sensed AV delay) can be programmed differently from the interval between a paced atrial and paced ventricular event (paced AV delay). The sensed AV delay is often empirically programmed shorter than the paced AV delay by about 30 msec to account for slower conduction through the atrium with pacing compared to spontaneous activation.

The AV delay can be programmed to mimic normal physiology, whereby the PR interval tends to shorten with exercise (shorter AV delay with a higher atrial rate—paced or sinus). In addition, shortening the AV delay improves the calculated URL for a pacemaker. The calculated URL is 60 seconds divided by the TARP, where TARP = AV interval + PVARP (see later). Thus, shortening the AV delay increases the calculated URL.

Importance of Minimizing Unnecessary Ventricular Pacing

Recent studies have shown that LBBB due to chronic right ventricular pacing may result in deterioration of left ventricular function when compared to a spontaneous narrow QRS without LBBB. Thus, impulses conducted through the AV node and the His-Purkinje system resulting in a narrow QRS would be expected to preserve left ventricular function better than constant ventricular pacing. For this reason, patients whose primary indication for pacemaker implantation is sinus node dysfunction should have long AV delays programmed in order to maximize the opportunity for impulse propagation through the normal conduction system. Because long AV delays compromise the URL, algorithms have been developed in permanent pacemakers to promote AAI pacing, with reversion to DDD if no ventricular activity is sensed after successive atrial-paced events. Such algorithms are not used in patients with advanced AV block, in whom ventricular pacing is obligatory. In these cases, shorter AV delays that allow an appropriate URL for the patient are employed.

Post Ventricular Atrial Refractory Period

The post ventricular atrial refractory period (PVARP) is the interval during which the atrial channel is blinded (refractory) to atrial activity. As the name indicates, this period starts after a sensed or paced ventricular event. The PVARP is designed to prevent retrograde P waves from being sensed and thus initiating another paced ventricular event, which can set up an endless loop tachycardia (ELT) or pacemaker-mediated tachycardia (PMT). An excessively long programmed PVARP is undesirable, because it will limit the calculated URL of the pacemaker (as just shown, URL = 60/AV + PVARP). Many pacemakers have automatic extension of the PVARP after a premature ventricular contraction (PVC), which allows programming of a more moderate PVARP during the majority of pacing while also minimizing the chances that ELT may be initiated after a PVC with retrograde conduction to the atrium.

Atrial and Ventricular Refractory Periods

The total atrial refractory period (or, as it is commonly abbreviated, TARP) is the sum of the AV delay and the PVARP. During the TARP, atrial activity that is detected by the atrial channel will be displayed as "AR" (for refractory atrial event) by the pacemaker programmer and is ignored for purposes of resetting timing or triggering ventricular pacing. Consequently, atrial activity that falls during the TARP will not be followed by paced ventricular activity. Atrial activity can only be tracked during the remaining part of the timing cycle.

The ventricular refractory period is the interval following a paced or sensed ventricular event during which spontaneous ventricular activity cannot be sensed. The purpose of this interval is to avoid T wave sensing or multiple sensing of ventricular activity due to delay in depolarization in different areas of the ventricles.

Blanking Periods and Crosstalk

The blanking period is an interval after an atrial output, whereby the ventricular channel is prevented from recognizing any electrical activity. This period is typically shorter than the ventricular refractory period and is usually about 10 to 50 msec. It is rarely necessary to reprogram blanking periods from nominal settings. The blanking period is designed to prevent crosstalk in dual-chamber pacemakers. Crosstalk occurs when the ventricular channel misinterprets the atrial output as ventricular activity, and consequently inhibits ventricular output. The result is ventricular asystole, which can be fatal in a pacemaker-dependent patient.

Upper Rate Behavior

In patients with DDD pacemakers, as the sinus rate increases, tracking of sinus activity results in 1:1 ventricular pacing up to the URL as defined by the TARP (**Table 7.4**). However, a 1:1 A:V relationship cannot be maintained in either of two circumstances: when the sinus rate exceeds the programmed URL despite the TARP being shorter than the URL, or when the TARP exceeds or is equal to the URL.

The first situation is shown in **Figure 7.2A**, in which the TARP is shorter than the interval for the programmed URL. In this patient, the sinus rate accelerates and ventricular pacing occurs after a fixed AV delay of 100 msec. In this pacemaker, the URL is programmed to 100 beats per minute (cycle length of 600 msec). The programmed AV delay is 100 msec and the PVARP is 300 msec, resulting in a TARP of 400 msec. As the sinus rate accelerates up to the URL (i.e., 100 beats/minute), 1:1 atrial tracking with ventricular pacing still occurs (see Figure 7.2A). When the sinus rate accelerates further to 115 beats per minute (above the URL), P waves still fall outside of PVARP. However, a 1:1 A:V response cannot occur because of the limiting URL. The P waves become progressively closer to the preceding paced ventricular beat

Table 7.4   Calculation of Upper Rate Limit
$URL = \dfrac{60{,}000 \text{ ms}}{TARP}$
TARP = AV interval + PVARP
PVARP = post ventricular atrial refractory period

(**Figure 7.2B**). When the P wave falls within the PVARP, no paced ventricular beat occurs (see the arrow in Figure 7.2B). Thus, a pattern of AV Wenckebach can be seen. This AV Wenckebach occurs because the sinus rate is faster than the programmed URL. This pattern of AV Wenckebach will persist until the sinus rate exceeds 150 beats per minute (60 seconds/TARP = 150 beats/min). If the sinus rate accelerates to 160 beats/minute (**Figure 7.2C**), every other sinus P wave will not be followed by a paced QRS, because it falls in the PVARP. Thus, 2:1 AV block occurs (see Figure 7.2C). From Figure 7.2, it can be seen that increasing sinus rates in the presence of TARP < URL lead to the development of pacemaker AV Wenckebach (see Figure 7.2B) followed by alternating P waves falling in the PVARP resulting in 2:1 AV block (see Figure 7.2C).

The second situation to consider occurs when the TARP is longer than the URL as illustrated in **Figure 7.3**. In this example, assume the AV interval is modified to 150 msec and the PVARP to 450 msec. Thus, TARP is now 600 msec, which is similar to the URL interval of 600 msec, unchanged from the previous programming. The maximum sinus rate that would result in 1:1 A:V conduction is 100 beats per minute, since the TARP is 600 msec and the calculated maximum rate is 60 s/600 ms, or 100 beats per minute (see **Figure 7.3A**). Further acceleration of the sinus rate would result in every other sinus P wave falling in the PVARP (arrows), resulting in 2:1 AV block (**Figure 7.3B**). Thus, when TARP > URL, 2:1 AV block occurs without being preceded by AV Wenckebach. Clinically, this may result in a patient reporting

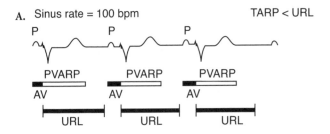

A. Sinus rate = 100 bpm   TARP < URL

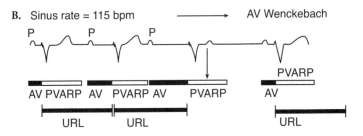

B. Sinus rate = 115 bpm   AV Wenckebach

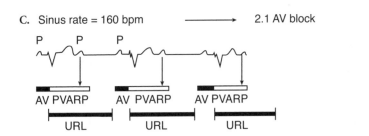

C. Sinus rate = 160 bpm   2.1 AV block

■ **Figure 7.2   Upper rate behaviors at various sinus rates when the TARP is less than the interval for the URL**

See text for details.

symptoms of sudden dizziness or fatigue during exercise, because of the sudden drop in the ventricular rate as the sinus rate is increasing. In the example given, the ventricular rate may drop suddenly from 100 beats per minute to about 50 beats per minute. In pacemaker programming, one will try to avoid sudden 2:1 AV block by keeping the TARP shorter than the URL.

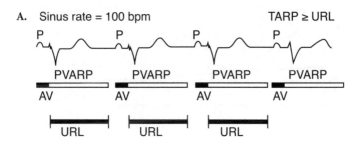

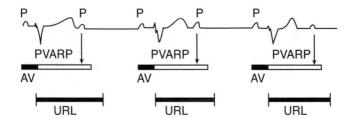

■ **Figure 7.3** **Upper rate behaviors at various sinus rates when TARP is equal to, or longer than, the interval for URL**

See text for details.

Clinical Factors to Consider in Pacemaker Programming

The programming of LRL, URL, AV delay, and PVARP are dictated by the patient's medical diagnosis, the pattern of retrograde conduction, and the patient's expectations. For example, a patient with severe coronary artery disease is probably better served by low LRL and URL (to avoid angina associated with high heart rates). On the other hand, a patient who expects to compete in sports will be better served by a higher URL, shorter AV delay, and shorter PVARP. A patient with a long V:A conduction time should have a reasonably long PVARP to minimize the possibility of PMT.

The choice of pacing mode, whether single chamber (VVI vs. AAI vs. VVIR vs. AAIR) or dual chamber (DDD vs. DDDR vs. VDD vs. DDI, etc.), will be influenced by factors such as atrial and ventricular EGM amplitudes, sinus node function, and the presence of intermittent or persistent AF, among others. For example, a patient with sinus rhythm and chronotropic incompetence will be better served by a DDDR pacemaker than a DDD pacemaker. To give another example, a patient with intermittent atrial flutter or AF, in whom automatic mode switching (AMS) (see Chapter 9) is not present or does not correctly detect atrial flutter or AF, may need to have the pacemaker programmed from the DDD to the DDI mode. A patient with a pacemaker showing a poor atrial pacing threshold may benefit from VDD rather than DDD pacing. In the great majority of pacemakers implanted today, a single-chamber pacemaker will have all potential single-chamber pacing modes programmable, and dual-chamber pacemakers likewise have all potential dual-chamber as well as single-chamber pacing modes programmable. Therefore, once one has made the decision as to whether a patient should have a single- or dual-chamber pacemaker implanted, the programmed pacing mode can be changed as necessary to meet the patient's needs.

Suggested Readings

Hayes DL. Timing cycles of permanent pacemakers. *Cardiol Clin.* 1992;10:593–608.

Hayes DL, Higano ST, Eisinger G. Electrocardiographic manifestations of a dual-chamber, rate-modulated (DDDR) pacemaker. *Pacing Clin Electrophysiol.* 1989;12:555–562.

Wilkoff BL, Cook JR, Epstein AE, et al. Dual-chamber pacing or ventricular backup pacing in patients with an implantable defibrillator. The Dual Chamber and VVI Implantable Defibrillator (DAVID) trial. *JAMA.* 2002;288:3115–3123.

8 ▪ Rate-Responsive Pacing

Cardiac pacemakers have always fulfilled the fundamental need for bradycardia rate support. In addition, triggering ventricular pacing after an atrial-sensed event restores AV synchrony in patients with AV block. In each case, however, a physiologic increase in heart rate with exercise is dependent on intact sinus node function. If the sinus node cannot respond to increasing metabolic demand, the result will be fixed-rate dual-chamber pacing. In the setting of AF with abnormal AV nodal conduction and a slow ventricular response, fixed-rate ventricular pacing will occur. The search for alternative means to increase pacing rate in such patients in response to increasing exercise demands led to the development of rate-responsive pacing.

Cardiac Output and Heart Rate

Cardiac output is the product of stroke volume and heart rate. While stroke volume may increase by approximately 50 percent with exercise, the heart rate may increase three- to fourfold in normal patients at peak exercise.

$$\text{Cardiac output} = \text{stroke volume} \times \text{heart rate}$$

Patients who cannot increase their heart rates with exercise are considered to have chronotropic incompetence. In such cases, pacemaker implantation will prevent pauses or bradycardia but will not restore exercise rate response. In order to do so in the setting of sinus node dysfunction, some other means of sensing the body's physiologic need for an increase in heart rate is necessary. Various sensors have been developed that have been incorporated into permanent pacemakers in order to meet this need.

The first rate-responsive pacemakers developed were single-chamber devices, mostly ventricular rate-responsive pacemakers, although some were used in the atrium for pure sinus node dysfunction. When patients with chronotropic incompetence undergo treadmill exercise testing and are tested with rate response on (VVIR pacing) versus off (VVI pacing), clear improvements in exercise time are observed. The difference between dual-chamber and single-chamber rate-responsive pacemakers in terms of exercise performance is much less marked, indicating that the atrial kick restored by dual-chamber pacing has a fairly minimal impact on exercise performance. In fact, AV synchrony is more important at rest and at low levels of exercise, while heart rate itself determines exercise performance at peak exertion. However, given what is now known about the detrimental effects of excessive ventricular pacing, an advantage of dual-chamber rate-responsive pacing is that ventricular pacing can be minimized in many patients with appropriate programming, while rate response is still provided.

Heart rate makes the greatest contribution to increasing cardiac output with exercise. It may increase up to fourfold, particularly in trained athletes, while stroke volume can only increase by about 50 percent.

Sensors

Sensors for rate-responsive pacing must detect some change in the body that correlates with increasing metabolic demand, and then translate that change into an increase in pacing rate (**Table 8.1**). Some of the most successful sensors for rate-responsive pacing, such as accelerometers, correlate imperfectly with metabolic demand. Others, such as body temperature, correlate quite well, but they have not been as successful in long-term development, for reasons that will be discussed later.

Motion-Based Sensors

There are two types of motion-based sensors: the activity sensor and the accelerometer. With the activity-based sensor, there is a piezoelectric crystal attached to the inside of the pacemaker can. It responds to body motion or vibration and is most sensitive to

Table 8.1   Sensors for Rate-Responsive Pacing

SENSOR	ADVANTAGES/DISADVANTAGES
Activity	Rapid response at initiation of exercise; may have elevated heart rates with vibration or other motion not related to exertion
Accelerometer	Rapid response at initiation of exercise; more responsive to forward motion than other types of exercise
Minute ventilation	Correlates well with oxygen consumption; slow to increase heart rate at the beginning of exercise
Evoked QT interval	Requires pacing for measurement; slow to increase heart rate at the beginning of exercise
Central venous temperature, pH, mixed venous oxygen saturation, etc.	Require special leads; not commercially available

up-and-down motion, as with the foot striking the ground. The accelerometer uses either a piezoelectric crystal or a piezoresistive unit mounted on the circuit board, and thus the sensor lies free within the pacemaker can. An accelerometer responds most to forward movement of the patient. One advantage of both of these types of technology is that the sensors are in the pacemaker generator itself, and thus special pacing leads are not required. With motion, signals are generated by the piezoelectric crystals. The frequency and amplitude of these signals are detected by the pacemaker generator, and an algorithm converts the current signal into a change in pacing rate. The simplicity of this approach is one of its strengths. However, body motion correlates only imperfectly with metabolic demand. For example, because an activity sensor will respond to any vibration, the more pronounced the vibration, the higher the pacing rate. Thus, patients who are walking downstairs, which causes a more pronounced striking of the foot on the stair, will have a higher pacing rate than when they are walking upstairs, even though the latter actually requires a higher heart rate physiologically. Other activities, such as riding in a car on a dirt road or working with a vacuum cleaner, could potentially elevate the heart rate inappropriately. Even tapping one's finger over the pacemaker generator is enough to increase the pacing rate.

The accelerometer, by virtue of the fact that it responds most sensitively to forward motion, may be less prone to excessive elevations of heart rate with pure vibratory motion. Regardless, both types of motion sensors have proven to be reliable and durable. In addition to simplicity and the ability to use a standard pacing lead, another advantage of motion-based sensors is that their response at the beginning of exercise is quite rapid. Heart rates quickly elevate to a level that will support increased activity by the patient.

> **Motion-based sensors for rate-responsive pacing are
> based on the piezoelectric crystal or a piezoresistive chip.
> The two types of motion sensors are the activity sensor and
> the accelerometer, which are distinguished by the location
> of the crystal within the pacemaker generator and the type of
> motion to which they respond.**

Minute Ventilation

The second most common type of sensor technology in permanent pacemakers is minute ventilation. Minute ventilation correlates closely with metabolic demand, and in fact, it increases almost linearly with heart rate during exercise. Changes in minute ventilation will change transthoracic impedance. In order to detect these changes, low amplitude, short-lived, constant current pulses are delivered at a rapid rate from the ring of the pacing lead to the pulse generator. Because the path of the current is through the thorax, impedance will vary as respiratory rate and tidal volume (the components of minute ventilation) change. This variation in impedance is detected by the pacemaker and converted into a change in pacing rate. The advantage of minute ventilation as a metabolic sensor is that it correlates very well with oxygen consumption. In addition, this sensor can be used with any standard bipolar pacing lead, because the sensor works simply by directing current pulses across the chest. A disadvantage of a minute ventilation sensor is that it is relatively slow to respond to changes in metabolic demand. Thus, the pacing rate does not increase as rapidly at the beginning of exercise as it should to mirror metabolic demand closely.

One way that this problem of slow response at onset of exercise with minute ventilation has been dealt with is by the development of blended sensors. In such systems, minute ventilation may be combined with an accelerometer or activity sensor. The motion sensors are set to control heart rate at the beginning of exercise, with minute ventilation being used as the primary sensor at peak exercise. These blended sensors require more complicated programming, and so they have not been used as widely as simple motion sensors.

Minute ventilation correlates well with metabolic demand, but the minute ventilation sensor does not respond as quickly at the beginning of exercise as motion sensors do.

QT Interval

The QT interval shortens with increasing heart rate, in response to sympathetic stimulation, as does the evoked, or paced, QT interval. This observation led to the development of evoked QT interval as a sensor for rate-responsive pacing. The advantage of this sensor, as with the ones just mentioned, is that only a standard pacing lead is required. The T wave after a paced complex is measured and pacing rate is varied according to an algorithm. Because QT interval shortening is less pronounced at low heart rates, algorithms have been developed to adjust the slope of the heart rate response to be steeper at low levels of exercise, with a decline in the slope as heart rate increases. Just as with minute ventilation, the evoked QT interval causes a slower rise in heart rate than is the case with motion sensors, but it is more proportional to metabolic demand. High impedance pacing leads, which can attenuate the T wave, are not suitable for use with evoked QT interval rate-responsive pacemakers.

Other Sensors

A number of other sensors have been studied for use in permanent pacemakers. However, none is available today in a commercially available pacemaker. The paced depolarization integral is one such sensor; it uses a standard pacing lead. The preejection interval, the time from the onset of ventricular depolarization to the onset of ventricular ejection, has also been investigated. Other sensors require special leads, which has limited their acceptance. Examples of such sensors include body temperature, pH, mixed venous oxygen saturation, and peak endocardial acceleration.

Despite the wide variety of sensors that have been investigated, the motion-based sensors remain the most popular in pacemaker generators. Simplicity of design and ease of programming have led to their widespread use over more than 20 years of rate-responsive pacing. Commercially available sensor combinations include activity and minute ventilation, and activity and QT interval.

Blended sensors, such as activity and minute ventilation, allow one to combine the advantages provided by each individual sensor for optimal exercise performance for the patient.

Programming

Upper Sensor Rate

A number of different parameters must be programmed in order to set up rate-responsive pacing for a patient (**Table 8.2**). First of all, it is necessary to program a lower pacing rate and an upper

Table 8.2   Programmed Parameters for Rate-Responsive Pacemakers

PARAMETER	USE
Upper sensor rate	Maximum pacing rate at peak activity
Threshold	Amount of activity that initiates sensor-based increase in heart rate
Slope	Change in pacing rate per unit change in sensor parameter
Acceleration	Speed of increase in heart rate at the beginning of exercise
Deceleration	Rate of decline in pacing rate after exercise ceases
Activities of daily living (ADL)	Rate expected for moderate activity, such as walking

pacing rate. In a single-chamber rate-responsive pacemaker (AAIR or VVIR), there is a single upper pacing rate that is programmed, and the actual pacing rate is determined by the sensor settings. In a dual-chamber rate-responsive pacemaker, it is possible to program separate upper *tracking* rates and *sensor* rates. The upper tracking rate means the upper rate that the pacemaker will pace in the ventricle based on the detected intrinsic sinus rate (atrial synchronous-ventricular pacing). Note that upper *tracking* rates are reached only in response to sinus tachycardia or some other spontaneous atrial tachyarrhythmia. If atrial pacing is occurring at rates above the base rate, then sensor-driven pacing is being observed. In a dual-chamber pacemaker, either ventricular pacing or spontaneous ventricular activation will occur in response to sensor-driven atrial pacing, up to the upper sensor rate. When both atrial sensing as well as the sensor-driven rate are dictating an increase in heart rate, the actual pacing rate will be whichever of the two rates is faster.

The upper sensor rate should be chosen based on a patient's age, medical condition, and normal activity level. A nominal upper rate of 120 beats per minute might be appropriate for a sedentary, elderly individual, but it could compromise exercise performance in someone younger or more active.

> **Upper sensor rates and tracking rates are independently programmable in dual-chamber pacemakers. In single-chamber pacemakers, there is only a single upper pacing rate based on the response to the sensor.**

Threshold

A second parameter that is programmed in rate-responsive pacing is the threshold for rate response. Typical settings would be low to high, with gradations in between, or numerical values from least sensitive to most sensitive. The best way to think of threshold is a bar at different heights, and one has to reach or exceed the bar to initiate an increase in pacing rate. Thus, a low threshold would indicate that mild activity would increase the pacing rate. It might be suitable for a fairly sedentary person, but there is also the risk of elevation in pacing rate out of proportion to the body's need because the sensor is set at an excessively sensitive setting. Medium-low and medium thresholds, or comparable numerical settings, are appropriate for most patients. Some models have auto-adjusting threshold levels that can be programmed on. In such cases, the pacemaker records activity levels over time, and then adjusts the threshold level to ensure that higher pacing rates will be reached about 1 percent of the time.

> **Threshold is the amount of activity that results in sensor detection to elevate heart rate. Low settings cause activity sensing with minimal activity and lead to rapid elevation of pacing rate, while the opposite is true for higher settings.**

Slope

Slope is always a parameter programmed in rate-responsive pacing. It dictates the rate of change in the pacing rate as the sensor-detected activity level increases. A very shallow slope can mean that, even though a patient has a high maximum sensor rate programmed, for all practical purposes it will never be reached as the patient exercises. On the other hand, a very steep slope means that a patient's heart rate will quickly reach the maximum pacing rate, even near the beginning of exercise when metabolic demands are modest. Moderate settings are best for most patients initially, and they can be adjusted in follow-up based on rate histogram profiles and the patient's symptoms. Many pacemakers now have a "redraw" feature that allows one to see how different rate response settings would affect the range of heart rates a patient achieves, as shown in **Figure 8.1**.

Slope dictates the rate of change in pacing rate with increasing activity levels.

Acceleration and Deceleration

Acceleration is another parameter that can be programmed to dictate what the change in pacing rate will be at the beginning of exercise, independent of the pure sensor-driven rate. Adjusting this parameter may be useful if a quicker heart rate response at the beginning of exercise is desired. Deceleration refers to the decline in pacing rate that occurs at the end of exercise. In any patient with a normal sinus node, heart rate returns gradually to normal at the end of exercise, with variations in the speed with which that happens depending on the patient's physical conditioning. In a patient with a permanent pacemaker, a rapid decline in pacing rate would not be physiologic and could lead to symptoms at the end of exercise. Programming the deceleration, or the period of time over

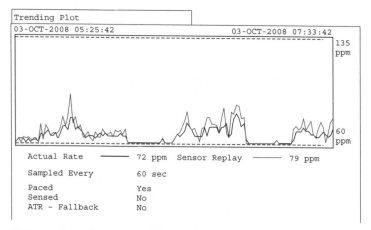

Trending Replay Parameters

	Present	Replay	
Lower Rate Limit	60	60	ppm
Max Sensor Rate	135	135	ppm
AutoLifestyle	Off	– –	
Accelerometer	On	On	
Activity Threshold	Medium	Med-Lo	
Reaction Time	30	30	sec
Response Factor	8	10	
Recovery Time	2	2	min
Minute Ventilation	On	On	
Response Factor	4	5	
High Rate Response Factor	55	55	%
High Rate Break Point	105	105	ppm

Trending Plot

03-OCT-2008 05:25:42   03-OCT-2008 07:33:42

135 ppm

60 ppm

Actual Rate	———	72 ppm	Sensor Replay	———	79 ppm

Sampled Every	60 sec
Paced	Yes
Sensed	No
ATR – Fallback	No

■ Figure 8.1   Rate response programming

The present programmed parameters for a dual-chamber rate-responsive pacemaker are shown on the top. The pacemaker has a blended sensor using both an accelerometer and minute ventilation. The "trending replay" on the bottom allows one to determine how changes in programmed parameters, in this case activity threshold and response factor, or slope, would affect the heart rates achieved with activity. The actual heart rates achieved with activity are shown in black, and the replay with the proposed new parameters are shown in gray.

which pacing rate returns to baseline, is a means of mimicking this natural decline in heart rate.

Activities-of-Daily-Living Rate

The activities-of-daily-living (ADL) rate is the heart rate one expects with moderate daily activities, such as walking. Commonly, it is programmed to values such as 90 to 100 beats per minute. When programmed on, it is another means of determining the degree of change in heart rate with various activities. With at least some pacemakers, the ADL rate will occur over a mid-range of sensor-detected activity counts, such that the heart rate slope will have a flat portion or plateau with moderate activity.

Calculated or Predicted Rate Profiles

One way to determine if the patient's current rate-responsive settings are adequate, besides assessment of symptoms such as exercise tolerance, is to analyze rate histograms. In a reasonably active patient, the majority of recorded heart rates will be near the LRL of the pacemaker, but there will also be a range of higher heart rates (see Chapter 10). If the histogram does not appear to be adequate, sensor settings may be adjusted, but it may take a return visit by the patient to determine how well they have worked to shift the pacing rates to a more physiologic range. An alternative approach to programming the sensor is available in some models of rate-responsive pacemakers. These models allow the clinician to see a graph displayed of heart rate variations with certain sensor settings. If the response does not appear to be adequate, it is possible to use a feature called the "calculated rate profile," or something similar, in which the graph can be redrawn by the software based on what would have been seen with alternative sensor settings (see Figure 8.1). It is thus possible to get a fairly good idea how the patient would respond to new settings immediately, allowing for further adjustment if necessary even before the patient leaves the clinic.

Many pacemakers now have the capability of automatic or semiautomatic programming of rate-response settings. Each manufacturer has its own terminology for the proprietary algorithm. In any case, when using such automatic programming, it is always important to review the resulting rate profiles when patients return to the clinic, ask about exercise tolerance, and make adjustments when necessary.

Suggested Readings

Clementy J, Barold S, Garrigue S, et al. Clinical significance of multiple sensor options: Rate response optimization, sensor blending, and trending. *Am J Cardiol.* 1999;83:166D–171D.

Shaber JD, Fisher JD, Ramachandra I, et al. Rate responsive pacemakers: A rapid assessment protocol. *Pacing Clin Electrophysiol.* 2008;31:192–197.

Strobel JS, Kay GN. Programming of sensor driven pacemakers. *Cardiol Clin.* 2000;18:157–176.

9 ■ Advanced Programming

ROBERT J. HARIMAN, MD, AND ANNE B. CURTIS, MD

There are a number of advanced programming features available in permanent pacemakers that may be applied in order to improve a patient's clinical status and/or prolong the pacemaker battery life. Certain functions are not available in all pacemakers. Some features are even proprietary to specific pacemaker manufacturers. Therefore, it is wise to anticipate the need for these functions before one decides to implant one type of pacemaker from a certain pacemaker manufacturer. Not infrequently, consultation with the technical support of the pacemaker manufacturer or the pacemaker company's representatives is advisable.

Automatic Mode Switching

AMS is a pacemaker function that is designed to prevent tracking of atrial activity during rapid atrial arrhythmias. For example, in a simple DDD or DDDR pacemaker without AMS, AF, which may be sensed by the atrial channel as atrial rates over 200 bpm, would trigger the ventricular channel to pace at the programmed URL. Ventricular pacing at the URL for a long period of time may cause symptoms and serious hemodynamic consequences. The ability to program AMS in dual-chamber pacemakers allows the benefit of AV synchrony when the patient is in normal sinus rhythm or a slow atrial rhythm, while AMS changes the pacemaker mode to a nonatrial tracking mode—VVI(R) or DDI(R)—during episodes of atrial tachyarrhythmias. The result is slower ventricular pacing, either at the LRL of the pacemaker or at the sensor-determined rate for AMS with VVIR or DDIR programming (**Figure 9.1**).

In addition, AMS data can be evaluated to determine the duration and frequency of AF episodes in a particular patient, as well as total AF burden (the duration of time in AF compared to the total duration of the monitoring period). This information, in

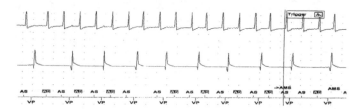

■ Figure 9.1   AMS

The elevated atrial rate is shown as multiple "AS" (atrial sensed) events. Those in the black boxes fall in the PVARP. Note that when AMS is triggered near the end of the recording, the ventricular pacing rate immediately begins to slow down.

turn, can be used as a tool in making the decision to anticoagulate a patient for the prevention of stroke.

> **The ability to program AMS in dual-chamber pacemakers allows the benefit of AV synchrony when the patient is in normal sinus rhythm or a slow atrial rhythm, with a change to a nonatrial tracking mode—VVI(R) or DDI(R)—during episodes of atrial tachyarrhythmias.**

Ideally, AMS should provide a high sensitivity and specificity for detecting atrial tachyarrhythmias (most commonly AF), minimize triggering of ventricular pacing at the URL, and restore AV synchrony when the atrial tachyarrhythmia ceases. Three factors that determine the AMS function should be considered:

1. Programmed parameters for atrial tachyarrhythmia detection
2. AMS response algorithm
3. Arrhythmia characteristics that may affect AMS behavior

Programming for Detection of Atrial Tachyarrhythmias
The programmed parameters that tell the pacemaker how to decide whether an atrial tachyarrhythmia is occurring are highly dependent on atrial sensing. Atrial sensing may be complicated by

smaller atrial EGMs that are often seen with AF compared to sinus rhythm; these smaller atrial EGMs may fall below the programmed atrial sensing level and thus may not be detected. Undersensing may also occur when atrial EGMs fall during the AV interval or the PVARP (during TARP) (see Chapter 7). Programming atrial sensitivity to avoid detection of far-field R waves and other signals not due to atrial depolarization is essential and must be considered when setting the sensitivity of the atrial channel.

In detecting an atrial tachyarrhythmia, AMS can be triggered by a certain length of time or a certain number of cycles of the atrial tachyarrhythmia. A rapid response of AMS requiring a short length of time or small number of short atrial cycles can lead to rate instability (rate oscillation), whereas a slow response can lead to long periods of ventricular pacing at the URL. There are two commonly used methods for a pacemaker to recognize an atrial tachyarrhythmia:

1. The most popular criterion is the rate cut-off. Sensed atrial rates exceeding a programmable value (for example, 170 bpm) for a defined period of time or a number of cycles shorter than a certain cycle length (for example, 353 msec) will trigger AMS. This algorithm provides fast onset of AMS and fast return to synchronized pacing. However, it may cause rapid oscillations of ventricular rates during the onset and offset of AMS.

2. The second algorithm uses running average rates, which are average rates that include the atrial activity during sinus rhythm. This algorithm continuously calculates the mean atrial rate. When the average rate gradually reaches the AMS trigger rate, AMS is activated. A gradual process in arriving at, and getting out of, the AMS trigger rate results from this AMS algorithm. This algorithm provides a more stable rate during AMS at the expense of a slower onset of AMS and a slower return to synchronized pacing.

> **The two most commonly used algorithms for detection of atrial tachyarrhythmias are rate cut-off and running average algorithms. The rate cut-off algorithm provides fast onset and offset of AMS at the expense of rapid oscillations of ventricular rates. The running average algorithm provides more stable ventricular pacing rates, but with slower onset of AMS and a slower return to synchronized pacing.**

The detection of atrial activity during TARP is a challenge. Therefore, in the rate cut-off algorithm, not all atrial cycle lengths are able to meet the cycle-length criterion (as in the previous example, 353 msec or a rate of 170 bpm), because some EGMs fall during the TARP. Therefore, in programming the rate cut-off criterion for AMS, the trigger for AMS will be satisfied, for example, when four of seven cycles fulfill the cycle length criterion, not seven of seven cycles.

AMS Response

In some pacemakers, different rates can be programmed during the mode switch. Thus, a period of time with a higher ventricular pacing rate at the onset of AMS can be selected to compensate for the loss of AV synchrony. In addition, rate responsiveness can be added during AMS, even if rate responsiveness is not programmed at times when AMS is not activated.

AMS algorithms also govern the time latency or the number of cycles needed to restore AV synchronous pacing after the atrial tachyarrhythmia terminates. In addition, rate-smoothing algorithms may be programmed for the period before the AMS rate becomes effective and during the return to AV synchrony. Thus, the change in ventricular pacing rate during activation of AMS can be made less abrupt by rate-smoothing algorithms, whereby a cap of a certain percentage (for example, 6%) is placed on beat-to-beat differences in cycle lengths. Rate smoothing thus prevents abrupt rate decreases when the pacemaker function changes from DDD with ventricular pacing at the URL (for example, 120 bpm) to VVI or DDI pacing due to AMS with ventricular pacing at 60 or 70 bpm. Rate smoothing may also mitigate any abrupt rate changes during the return to AV synchrony.

Arrhythmia Characteristics and AMS Response

The type of atrial tachyarrhythmia and the nature of AV conduction may also complicate AMS. In general, AF with irregular and rapid atrial cycle lengths of less than 200 msec triggers AMS more readily, unless the atrial EGMs of the AF are below the sensitivity setting of the pacemaker. However, AMS detection of atrial flutter represents a challenge. Many patients with tachycardia due to atrial flutter and 2:1 AV block may fail to trigger AMS. This phenomenon is termed 2:1 lock-in. In 2:1 lock-in, every other atrial EGM falls during PVARP. To reliably detect atrial flutter in this situation, an "atrial flutter response" has been developed. When AMS is suspected, atrial flutter response leads to a change in PVARP and the ventricular pacing rate in order to expose the rapid atrial activity.

AMS has been used as a surrogate of AF occurrence and a measure of how well AF has been controlled. Thus, one can measure the time to the first occurrence of AMS, the frequency of the AMS, and the duration of the AMS. AF burden, which is defined as the proportion of time a patient is in AF, can be used as one factor in deciding whether a patient with paroxysmal AF should be placed on anticoagulation for stroke prevention.

> **Programmed values for detection of atrial tachyarrhythmias, characteristics of the AMS algorithm, and the nature of the tachyarrhythmia itself all factor into the response to AMS.**

In a randomized crossover study evaluating the symptomatic benefit of AMS, whereby patients with intermittent atrial tachyarrhythmias were randomized to dual-chamber pacing with AMS, dual-chamber pacing without AMS, and single-chamber pacing, patients reported symptomatic benefit in dual-chamber pacing with AMS. This benefit may be related to avoidance of tachycardia-related symptoms (due to rapid ventricular pacing during atrial tachyarrhythmias) and the ability to have synchronous pacing during slower atrial or sinus rhythms.

Autothreshold Function

Automatic testing for atrial or ventricular pacing threshold is commonly used today. Periodic capture testing and adjustment of output are important to ensure reliable pacemaker capture and to conserve battery life. Atrial and ventricular capture threshold testing is made possible through the use of a stimulation program with variation in pulse amplitude and width to check pacing threshold on a regular basis. Based on the results, the atrial and ventricular outputs are then automatically adjusted. The pacemaker will automatically program the output just above the capture threshold to preserve the battery life. This function is especially important in patients with unstable conditions that may affect the pacing threshold. These conditions include, for example, fluctuations of autonomic tone, serum potassium levels, arterial oxygen content, and antiarrhythmic drug levels. Myocardial ischemia or infarction can also increase pacing thresholds, potentially leading to ventricular noncapture. The autothreshold function can prevent this eventuality. A summary of advanced programming features in permanent pacemakers, including autothreshold, is provided in **Table 9.1**.

> **The autothreshold function varies pacing output on a regular basis, determines whether capture is adequate, and adjusts pacing output accordingly.**

Table 9.1 Advanced Programming Features in Permanent Pacemakers

FEATURE	DESCRIPTION
AMS	Automatic detection of atrial tachyarrhythmias with a change to a non-atrial tracking pacing mode
Autothreshold	Automatic measurement of pacing threshold and adjustment of pacing output
Autointrinsic conduction search	Periodic increase in AV interval to favor intrinsic AV conduction over ventricular pacing
Pacemaker-mediated tachycardia termination	Periodic extension of PVARP if conditions that indicate or favor development of PMT are met
Atrial overdrive pacing and others	Algorithms designed for suppression of atrial tachyarrhythmias
Rate hysteresis	Intrinsic rhythm allowed at rates lower than the programmed LRL
AV hysteresis	Intrinsic AV conduction permitted at AV intervals longer than programmed
Sleep rate	Lower pacing rate during night hours and/or during periods of inactivity as detected by a sensor
Rate-drop response	Temporary increase in pacing rate triggered by an abrupt drop in intrinsic heart rate

Autointrinsic Conduction Search

Constant apical right ventricular pacing has been shown to cause worsening of left ventricular function and congestive heart failure, presumably because apical right ventricular pacing causes cardiac desynchronization. Thus, in the DAVID (Dual-Chamber and VVI Implantable Defibrillator) trial (see also Chapter 7), patients with dual-chamber pacing had worsening of left ventricular function compared with patients who had ventricular depolarization from intrinsic AV conduction. In MOST (Mode Selection Trial), patients with sick sinus syndrome had increased rates of hospitalization when they had frequent apical right ventricular pacing. Thus, avoidance of constant apical right ventricular pacing is desirable, and there are a few options that a physician can choose to accomplish this. One option is programming to an atrial pacing mode (AAI or AAIR). However, it is well recognized that a small percentage (approximately 0.6% per year) of patients with sick sinus syndrome develops AV block. Alternatively, programming of a fixed, long AV delay may minimize ventricular pacing. However, as discussed in Chapter 7, this approach will prolong the TARP and reduce the effective URL for pacing. Recognizing the limitations of these options, some pacemakers now have algorithms that automatically search for intrinsic ventricular depolarizations. If there are no intrinsic ventricular depolarizations sensed within a preset long AV interval, ventricular pacing will resume at the programmed shorter AV delay. Using such algorithms, which go by names such as *autointrinsic conduction search* or *minimal ventricular pacing*, ventricular pacing is minimized and the URL for pacing is not jeopardized.

> **Algorithms for minimizing ventricular pacing can provide atrial pacing with monitoring of AV conduction and conversion to dual-chamber pacing if there is failure of intrinsic ventricular depolarization.**

Pacemaker-Mediated Tachycardia Termination Algorithms

PMT (also termed endless loop tachycardia or ELT) is an artificial reentrant tachycardia that can occur as a complication of dual-chamber pacing. In PMT, a ventricular depolarization (spontaneous or paced)is conducted retrogradely through the

AV node to the atria, causing atrial depolarization. This atrial depolarization is sensed by the atrial channel of the dual-chamber pacemaker, which then triggers the ventricular channel to pace the ventricles. Therefore, the pacemaker circuit senses atrial activity and triggers ventricular pacing; this sequence constitutes the anterograde limb of the PMT. The tachycardia perpetuates by repeated conduction of ventricular depolarizations to the atria, with sensing of the resulting atrial depolarization and repeated triggering of ventricular pacing. Thus, based on the previous sequence, development of PMT requires sensing of atrial activity (second letter of A or D in the pacemaker mode designation) and atrial triggering of ventricular pacing (third letter T or D). Therefore, pacemakers in the DDD, VDD, VAD, and VAT modes can be associated with PMT. Typically, the tachycardia rate during PMT is equal to the URL set for the dual-chamber pacemaker. The patient may complain of palpitations and other consequences of hypoperfusion during PMT.

Not all constant pacing at the URL of the pacemaker is due to PMT. Atrial tachyarrhythmias (sinus or atrial tachycardia, atrial flutter or AF) can trigger the ventricular channel to pace at the URL. In unipolar pacemakers, oversensing of myopotentials from the chest muscles can also trigger ventricular pacing at the URL. In the past, pacemaker circuitry malfunction could result in a "runaway pacemaker" with pacing at very high rates. In order for heart rates at the upper pacing rate of the pacemaker to be due to PMT, there must be a demonstrated artificial reentrant tachycardia. Retrieval of intracardiac EGMs showing lack of a 1:1 A:V relationship and lack of A-sense, V-trigger sequences and VA conduction would be inconsistent with PMT/ELT. Pacemaker interrogation showing the EGMs recorded by the atrial channel and the onset/termination of the tachycardia are helpful in the differentiation of these causes of ventricular pacing at the upper rate of the pacemaker.

In an acute situation, such as in the emergency room, applying a magnet over the pacemaker will disable atrial sensing (and also ventricular sensing). Because atrial sensing is disabled, triggering of ventricular pacing is not possible. Thus, a magnet basically eliminates the anterograde limb of the reentrant circuit in PMT. In addition, magnet application changes the pacing mode from DDD to DOO, which can lead to restoration of sinus rhythm after the magnet is removed. More permanent prevention of PMT is achieved by reprogramming of the pacemaker.

The main way to prevent PMT is the use of an appropriate length of the PVARP. If VA conduction is present during implantation of the pacemaker, PVARP should be made long enough so that retrograde atrial depolarization falls during the PVARP. There are potential limitations to this approach. First, some patients may exhibit intermittent VA conduction. For example, a patient may not have VA conduction during implantation, and yet under different conditions of autonomic tone, the patient may exhibit VA conduction and the ability to develop PMT. Second, a long PVARP prolongs the TARP and reduces the upper limit for atrial tracking (see Chapter 7). The common short-term approach to this problem is to keep the AV delay short and the PVARP long, since TARP = AV delay + PVARP.

Prevention of PMT is best accomplished by the use of an appropriate duration of PVARP.

From this discussion, it is apparent that prolongation of the PVARP has limitations. Therefore, many pacemaker manufacturers have developed various proprietary algorithms for termination of PMT. Because premature ventricular beats with retrograde conduction to the atria are a common cause of PMT, a typical algorithm involves temporary prolongation of the PVARP when a premature ventricular beat is recognized by the pacemaker. This algorithm allows a shorter PVARP for other beats.

Modern pacemakers have incorporated other algorithms to terminate an ongoing PMT. For example, the pacemaker can be programmed to extend the PVARP of every ninth paced ventricular beat during ventricular pacing at the URL (which is suggestive of PMT). This algorithm may cause intermittent non-sensing during sinus tachycardia. Other more complex ways to prevent and terminate PMT have been developed. One of them is termed *differential atrial sensing*. In this algorithm, if retrograde atrial depolarization is smaller in amplitude than anterograde atrial depolarization, the pacemaker can be programmed to ignore (not sense) retrograde atrial activity, while still sensing anterograde atrial activity. However, the assumption that retrograde atrial activity is smaller than anterograde atrial activity is not always correct.

The approach to a pacemaker patient with intermittent tachycardia involves retrieving the EGMs during the tachycardia. If PMT is suspected, the AV delay should be shortened, while the PVARP is lengthened. Automatic PVARP extension for premature ventricular beats and automatic intermittent PVARP extension during ventricular pacing at the URL may be applied. In patients with suspected PMT, physicians usually reduce the URL to about 100 bpm in order to prevent symptomatic tachycardia, until they are certain that PMT has been corrected. The atrial pacing threshold should also be assessed, since atrial noncapture with ventricular pacing and subsequent retrograde atrial depolarization can provide the substrate for PMT. Sometimes, certain functions like autointrinsic conduction search will make the AV delay long and the PVARP short. This complicates the approach to treating patients with PMT. One may decide to eliminate this function until the PMT problem is solved.

PVARP programming, PVARP extension after a PVC or at periodic intervals when the pacemaker is pacing the ventricles at the upper pacing rate, as well as differential atrial sensing, are approaches that may be used to prevent PMT.

Algorithms for Suppression and Termination of Atrial Tachyarrhythmias

Some pacemakers have algorithms designed to pace the atrium at a rapid rate when frequent atrial ectopic beats in succession occur. The intention is to overdrive pace the atrial ectopic beats and reduce dispersion of atrial refractory periods so that these atrial ectopic beats do not degenerate into AF. Following the rapid atrial pacing, the pacing rate is reduced gradually to enable the pacemaker to look for baseline intrinsic atrial rhythm. The rapid pacing may be repeated at a higher rate, if necessary. As concluded by the Science Advisory Panel of the American Heart Association, for patients who have a bradycardia indication for pacing and also have AF, no consistent data from large randomized trials support the use of overdrive atrial pacing for prevention of atrial tachyarrhythmias, nor are there data to support the routine use of antitachycardia pacing (ATP) for the termination of atrial tachyarrhythmias. At present, it is unclear whether these pacing modalities are of any real value in the management of AF, and thus this aspect of pacing is still under development.

No consistent data from large randomized trials support the use of atrial overdrive or ATP for the prevention or termination of atrial tachyarrhythmias.

Hysteresis

Pacemakers can be programmed to have a longer escape interval (for example, 1,200 msec or a rate of 50 bpm) than the baseline pacing interval (for example, 857 msec or a rate of 70 bpm). This programming function is called positive rate hysteresis. The purpose of hysteresis is to try to keep patients in their intrinsic rhythm (usually sinus rhythm) as much as possible. The advantage of a spontaneous rhythm is the maintenance of AV synchrony (if there is normal AV conduction), with normal depolarization of the ventricles through the His-Purkinje system rather than dyssyn-chronous ventricular activation from right ventricular pacing.

In the example just given, the pacemaker will pace at 70 bpm until a spontaneous rhythm faster than 70 bpm occurs. Then pacing will be inhibited until the intrinsic rate drops below 50 bpm, after which pacing at 70 bpm will resume. In a more advanced algorithm, after a given number of pacing beats at 70 bpm, the pacemaker drops its rate to 50 bpm to look for any escape beats at intervals shorter than 1,200 msec (faster than 50 bpm). This function is called search hysteresis. Search hysteresis is activated periodically until spontaneous cardiac activity faster than the hysteresis rate occurs.

In addition to rate hysteresis, there is a less commonly used hysteresis function that affects the AV delay. Positive AV interval hysteresis results in prolongation of the AV delay after a determined number of atrial beats to look for spontaneous AV conduction. This function has the same goal as the autointrinsic conduction search. Negative AV interval hysteresis is used mainly for hypertrophic cardiomyopathy with the intention of ensuring ventricular capture with a short AV delay. During stress, the intrinsic AV delay may shorten, so a negative AV interval hysteresis ensures ventricular capture. This function is not commonly used because of its limited indication.

Rate hysteresis may lead to some otherwise unexpected pacing behaviors, such as lack of pacing during sinus rhythm at 60 bpm when the pacing rate is 70 bpm.

Sleep Rates

Modern pacemakers can be programmed to a slower pacing rate during sleep. It is expected that metabolic activities are reduced during sleep and slower heart rates are more compatible with a better sleep. Therefore, a pacemaker can be programmed to have a slower rate (for example, 50 bpm) during sleep while a faster rate (for example, 70 bpm) is programmed during waking hours. There are two ways that are being used to synchronize this function with the sleeping time. First, the pacemaker can be programmed to have a slower pacing rate during certain hours (for example, from 10:00 PM to 6:00 AM). Alternatively, some pacemakers can be programmed to activate the sleep pacing rate when the activity sensor (the piezoelectric crystal) detects lack of activity. There is also an algorithm that requires both criteria to be met before the sleep rate is activated.

Rate-Drop Response

Rate-drop response is a programming feature that is used for the management of neurocardiogenic syncope. As discussed in Chapter 3, recurrent neurocardiogenic syncope is only a class IIb indication for pacing. If it is used at all, pacing should be most helpful in the patient with a prominent cardioinhibitory (bradycardia or asystole) component during episodes. The recommended pacing mode for neurocardiogenic syncope is either DDD or DDI in order to maintain AV synchrony and the atrial kick during symptomatic episodes. With rate-drop response, a sudden decrease in heart rate triggers an elevated pacing rate for a programmed period of time (several minutes), after which the pacing rate drops back gradually to the baseline rate. For example, the trigger for the temporary pacing rate could be a lengthening of the R-R cycle length for at least two or more consecutive beats by a certain percentage (such as 40%) or a drop in heart rate to a certain level (for example, 40 bpm). The reason for the requirement of two or more consecutive beats with a long cycle length is to avoid triggering this function by premature ventricular beats with a compensatory pause. After dual-chamber pacing has been instituted for the programmed length of time, hysteresis can be used to search for restoration of the spontaneous baseline heart rate to determine if bradycardia is still present.

Rate-drop response is a programming feature available in some dual-chamber pacemakers that is used for the management of selected patients with neurocardiogenic syncope. It results in an elevated pacing rate for several minutes if an abrupt drop in heart rate is detected.

Suggested Readings

Connolly SJ, Sheldon R, Roberts RS, Gent M. The North American Vasovagal Pacing Study. A randomized trial of permanent cardiac pacing for the prevention of vasovagal syncope. *Am Coll Cardiol.* 1999;33:21–23.

Kamalvand K, Tan K, Kotsakis A, et al. Is mode switching beneficial: A randomized study in patients with atrial tachyarrhythmias. *J Am Coll Cardiol.* 1997;30:496–504.

Knight BP, Gersh BJ, Carlson MD, et al. Role of permanent pacing to prevent atrial fibrillation: Science advisory from American Heart Association Council on Clinical Cardiology (Subcommittee on Electrocardiography and Arrhythmias) and the Quality of Care and Outcomes Research Interdisciplinary Working Group, in Collaboration with the Heart Rhythm Society. *Circulation.* 2005;111:240–243.

Sweeney MO, Hellkamp AS, Ellenbogen KA, et al. Adverse effect of ventricular pacing on heart failure and atrial fibrillation among patients with normal baseline QRS duration in a clinical trial of pacemaker therapy for sinus node dysfunction. *Circulation.* 2003; 23:2932–2937.

10 ■ Diagnostics

Pacemakers have a variety of diagnostics that can be extremely helpful in device follow-up, including assessment of pacemaker function and the detection and diagnosis of arrhythmias. A brief description of the most common types of diagnostics is provided in this chapter; their value will become evident in Chapter 12. It should be noted that each of the pacemaker manufacturers has slight variations in the terminology of the different possible diagnostic features and the way the data are collected and displayed (**Table 10.1**).

Battery Status

Information on battery voltage, battery impedance, and current drain are routinely provided when a pacemaker is interrogated. As discussed in Chapter 5, the battery in a pacemaker generator has 2.8 V when it is first implanted. The battery current drain reflects the current being drawn from the battery as pacing outputs are provided over time, in addition to the minimal current drain that occurs when the pacemaker is relatively quiescent. Because the pacemaker battery has a known capacity of microampere-hours, the measured current drain can be used to calculate the remaining longevity of the battery. Changes in pacing rate or output can markedly affect the projected longevity of the battery.

Battery impedance is inversely related to battery voltage. As lithium iodide is generated by the chemical reaction in the lithium-iodine battery, it forms a resistive barrier between the cathode and the anode. This chemical accumulation increases the internal impedance of the battery.

Upon interrogation of a pacemaker, there will be information available on battery voltage, current, and impedance and usually some calculation of the remaining longevity of the battery. This

Table 10.1   Diagnostic Features in Permanent Pacemakers

FEATURE	USE
Battery status	Assess remaining longevity of battery; battery impedance and current drain also reported.
Impedance monitoring	Assess integrity of pacing lead.
Pacing threshold monitoring	Automatically assess pacing threshold and adjust output to maintain capture. Graphs of trends over time can help to detect early lead failure.
Sensing threshold monitoring	Assess sensed signals and adjust sensing threshold as necessary; may switch polarity if necessary.
Event counters	Determine percentages of atrial and ventricular pacing and sensing; most useful for adjustment of AV intervals if percent ventricular pacing is high.
Rate histograms	Determine whether rate response should be programmed, or if already in use, whether the response is adequate.
High atrial rate episodes	Assess the presence and duration of atrial tachyarrhythmias.
Mode switch episodes	Record the number of times the pacemaker has switched to a non-atrial tracking mode in response to atrial tachyarrhythmias.
Event markers	Diagnose arrhythmias and assess pacemaker behavior by comparing EGM/ECG data to sensed and paced events from the pacemaker.

information may be presented as an estimate of the number of years of battery life remaining, or as a graph showing present battery status compared to BOS and EOS (**Figure 10.1**).

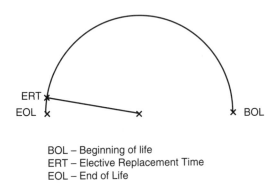

	Previous	Present
Date of last test	18-JUL-2008	
Battery Status	ERT	ERT
Effective Magnet Rate	85	85
Time Since ERT	Set	08-JUL-2008

BOL – Beginning of life
ERT – Elective Replacement Time
EOL – End of Life

■ **Figure 10.1   Battery status display**

The patient's pacemaker generator has reached the elective replacement time (ERT).

> **As battery voltage declines, internal impedance increases.**
> **Interrogation of the pacemaker to determine the present values**
> **of voltage and impedance provides information on the**
> **remaining battery life before generator change will be necessary.**

Impedance Monitoring

Measurement of pacing lead impedance is an important means of determining the integrity of the pacing lead. Note that this impedance is distinct from the impedance of the battery. Pacing lead impedance is measured at the time of lead implantation and at every follow-up visit. In addition, most pacemakers today track lead impedance over time, and they can provide a graph of trends in lead impedance (**Figure 10.2**). Impedance is usually stable within a narrow range of values. Marked variability in lead impedance is evidence of a lead or set screw problem, while a significant increase or decrease in lead impedance can be evidence of lead fracture or a disruption in the insulation, respectively. It is important to note that stability of the impedance value for an individual lead is more important than the specific impedance value itself. For example, a lead with an impedance of 400 ohms is inherently not more or less stable than a lead with an impedance of 800 ohms. However, if the lead with an impedance of 800 ohms suddenly measures 400 ohms, this change can be an indication of a problem with the lead insulation. The lead monitor feature of modern pacemakers also allows the pacemaker to automatically switch pacing and sensing polarity from bipolar to unipolar if high- or low-pacing impedances are detected.

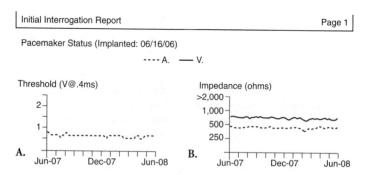

■ **Figure 10.2   Threshold and lead impedance trends**

A. Threshold trend. Atrial pacing threshold is stable at approximately 0.7 V over time.

B. Lead impedance. Both atrial and ventricular lead impedances are stable over time.

A marked change in pacing impedance, either higher or lower, is more important in diagnosing a potential problem with a pacing lead than the absolute value of the impedance itself.

Threshold Monitoring

Just as with impedance monitoring, long-term pacing threshold monitoring is available in many newer model pacemakers (see Figure 10.2). In order to have this kind of data available from a pacemaker, the generator must be capable of automatically checking pacing thresholds on a regular basis and adjusting pacing outputs accordingly. Particularly with the widespread use today of steroid-eluting leads, there usually is fairly minimal deterioration in pacing thresholds from the time of implantation to the initial follow-up visit. After that, pacing thresholds tend to be stable over time. Unfavorable trends in pacing threshold tend to parallel changes in lead impedance, so that marked increases or decreases in impedance will often be associated with increases in pacing threshold.

In addition to automatic pacing threshold monitoring, many pacemakers have an automatic sensing threshold feature. The peak amplitude of the sensed signal is measured and sensitivity is automatically increased or decreased to maintain an adequate safety margin.

Pacemakers that are programmed to automatically check pacing threshold and adjust output accordingly can provide long-term pacing threshold trends, which can be used in conjunction with impedance trends to monitor the status of pacing leads.

Event Counters

Some of the most important information that can be obtained from interrogation of a pacemaker is the distribution of paced and sensed events and the distribution of heart rates for these different combinations. For example, there are four combinations of events that can be counted. The first is atrial-sensed, ventricular-sensed events, which is simply the pacemaker's terminology for the intrinsic, usually sinus, rhythm. The notation for these events may be AS-VS, or alternatively, P-R, depending on the manufacturer. Other combinations include atrial pacing with ventricular sensing (AP-VS, or A-R), atrial sensing with ventricular pacing (AS-VP, or P-V), or atrial pacing with ventricular pacing (AP-VP, or A-V). The percentage of time spent in each of these different combinations of pacing and sensing is displayed with the pacemaker interrogation, either as individual percentages or as bar graphs as well. High percentages of ventricular pacing can be an indication that the programmed AV delay should be reviewed and extended, if doing so is likely to increase the percentage of spontaneous ventricular activation (i.e., advanced AV block is not present). In addition to percentages of time in the different paced and sensed configurations, information on other arrhythmias such as PVCs is often available. PVCs will be counted when ventricular-sensed events occur with no associated atrial activity.

Event counters will provide information on the percentage of time there is atrial sensing or pacing and ventricular sensing or pacing. Review of the information can help to determine how much pacing is being provided and whether programmed AV delays need to be adjusted.

Rate Histograms

In addition to assessment of a patient's symptoms and exercise tolerance, rate histograms are used in conjunction with the event counters to determine whether changes in programmed rates are advisable. A typical patient spends most of his or her time at lower heart rates, because of the amount of time spent sleeping or in sedentary pursuits. There should be a range of heart rates above that, tapering off at heart rates near the maximum exercise rate.

This range of heart rates is usually displayed in a histogram, showing the relative percentage of time the patient spends in each 10-beat increment in heart rate. In addition, the percentage of time that is paced versus sensed is displayed, with separate histograms for atrial and ventricular activity (**Figure 10.3**).

Rate histograms that show all or nearly all heart rates at the lower pacing rate of the pacemaker are an indication that rate response should be activated, if it has not been already, or that the settings are too conservative. Conversely, if a patient is able to mount a normal increase in sinus rate with activity, as shown by sensed heart rates at higher levels, rate response may not even be necessary. In addition, an assessment of sensed versus paced activity may indicate whether programmed AV intervals should be lengthened, if spontaneous conduction is possible, or even shortened if there is no intrinsic AV conduction and longer AV intervals may compromise the upper pacing rate that can be achieved.

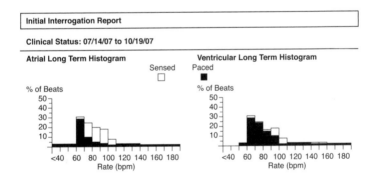

■ Figure 10.3   Atrial and ventricular rate histograms

At the LRL, the patient is paced in both chambers nearly 100% of the time. The histograms show that the sinus rate increases spontaneously, since higher atrial rates are mainly sensed and not paced. The ventricle is paced the great majority of the time, indicating either that the patient has advanced AV block or that the AV delay has been programmed shorter than the spontaneous conduction time.

Rate histograms are extremely helpful in determining whether a patient has a normal heart rate range during spontaneous sinus rhythm, or alternatively, whether rate-responsive pacing settings provide an adequate range of heart rates with daily activities.

Atrial High-Rate Episodes

Dual-chamber pacemakers can provide a wealth of information on the number of atrial high-rate episodes, their duration, including the shortest and longest episodes, and overall AF "burden," defined as the amount of time spent in AF compared to sinus rhythm or normal atrial pacing. The term "atrial high rate" is a means of communicating that rapid atrial rates have been detected, without automatically labeling them with a specific diagnosis. The heart rate over which high rates are counted is programmable, and it should be programmed differently in young individuals compared to older patients.

The counters and date/time stamps for atrial high-rate episodes and other diagnostics are memory intensive, and so it is not realistic to expect unlimited information in this regard in current pacemakers. Usually, there are a specific number of episodes that can be recorded before the counters are "saturated" and no further information will be recorded until the counters are cleared. Alternatively, if the memory becomes filled, recording of newer information may cause the oldest data to be erased. For these reasons, it is important to download information on diagnostics at the time of pacemaker interrogation and to clear the counters before the patient leaves the office, in order to be able to record new data in follow-up. Another reason for clearing out the counters is so that when a patient returns to the clinic, the information downloaded is the most recent information on patient activity and heart rates, and it is not obscured by old data that has not been saved and then erased.

In addition to the dates, times, and durations of atrial high-rate episodes, at least some EGM data is stored from some of the episodes, such as the longest. Review of these EGMs will allow the clinician to determine whether the episode was indeed due to an elevated atrial rate. For example, if far-field R waves are detected in addition to P waves, the recorded atrial rate will be twice the actual heart rate. On the other hand, rapid atrial rates may be due to atrial flutter or AF that may be easily recognized by review of the intracardiac EGMs during the event.

With review of atrial high-rate episodes, it may become apparent that a patient is having episodes of paroxysmal AF. If so, it may be necessary to review the patient's risk factors for thromboembolism according to the congestive heart failure/hypertension/age > 75 years/diabetes mellitus/previous stroke or transient ischemic attack ($CHADS_2$) score and consider whether anticoagulation with warfarin is warranted. An interesting dilemma is what duration and/or frequency of apparent AF episodes should lead to anticoagulation in an asymptomatic patient; there is currently no consensus in this regard.

Atrial high-rate episodes provide information on the number and duration of episodes of elevated atrial rates that exceed a programmable threshold. AF burden refers to the total amount of time spent in AF compared to the total duration of monitoring time.

Mode-Switch Episodes

As discussed in Chapter 9, mode switching is a feature whereby detection of atrial rates that exceed a programmable level leads to a change in pacing mode to a nontracking mode, such as DDD/DDDR to DDI/DDIR. The diagnostic for mode-switch episodes records the number of times that mode switching has occurred along with the date and time. The rates detected during mode-switch episodes should be reviewed, along with the intracardiac EGMs where available, to ensure that the mode switching is occurring for true atrial tachyarrhythmias for which tracking is undesirable. Nominal settings for mode switching are usually around 175 beats per minute, which exceeds the upper sinus rate of most patients who receive permanent pacemakers. If mode switching is seen to occur for sinus tachycardia, the programmed mode-switch rate should be increased. As with atrial high-rate episodes, frequent mode-switch episodes should lead to initiation of systemic anticoagulation in appropriate patients. In addition, it may be prudent to consider whether other drug therapy, such as AV nodal blockers or antiarrhythmic drugs, should be started or doses adjusted.

Frequent mode switching, if it is confirmed to be due to recurrent supraventricular tachyarrhythmias, may require a reevaluation of a patient's medical therapy, particularly the use and dosage of antiarrhythmic drugs.

Event Markers

Event markers provide information on real-time pacing system behavior as interpreted by the pacemaker. The terminology varies from manufacturer to manufacturer and may be called marker channels, main timing events, or annotated event markers. The information is most valuable when displayed simultaneously with a surface ECG. Multichannel recordings may allow display of intracardiac atrial and/or ventricular EGMs as well. In addition to annotations such as "AS" for an atrial-sensed event or "R" for a sensed R wave, timing intervals for event markers are provided by some manufacturers. It should be noted that event markers provide information as to how the pacemaker interprets sensed signals and what outputs are occurring. Sensed signals are not necessarily interpreted correctly by the pacemaker, and paced outputs do not necessarily result in capture. The clinician must interpret the event markers in conjunction with the EGMs and the ECG to determine if pacing behavior is normal. Examples of the use of event markers for troubleshooting are provided in Chapter 12.

Most event marker recordings are done "real time," by reviewing pacing behavior while the patient is being evaluated in clinic. It is now possible in some cases to store events along with event markers for later review. Such would be the case for a triggered event recording by a patient, or storage of events that meet certain predefined criteria. These recordings are memory intensive, so the number of such events is usually limited in number and duration.

Event markers provide annotations of pacing system behavior. They are extremely helpful in troubleshooting pacemaker problems when recorded in conjunction with a surface ECG lead and intracardiac atrial and ventricular EGMs.

Other Diagnostics

Other diagnostics that can be provided by many pacemakers include high ventricular rate episodes, sudden rate-drop episodes (for patients with neurocardiogenic syncope), the number of times a PMT algorithm was activated, and how long the pacemaker functioned at the URL, among others.

Suggested Readings

Nowak B. Taking advantage of sophisticated pacemaker diagnostics. *Am J Cardiol.* 1999;83(5B):172D–179D.

Nowak B, McMeekin J, Knops M, et al. Validation of dual-chamber pacemaker diagnostic data using dual-channel stored electrograms. *Pacing Clin Electrophysiol.* 2005;28:620–629.

Pollak WM, Simmons JD, Interian A Jr, et al. Pacemaker diagnostics: A critical appraisal of current technology. *Pacing Clin Electrophysiol.* 2003;26(1 Pt 1):76–98.

11 ■ Follow-Up

GUSTAVO LOPERA, MD, AND ANNE B. CURTIS, MD

The goals of the acute and long-term follow-up of patients with pacemakers are to optimize pacemaker function according to the patient's needs, recognize complications related to the pacing therapy, identify and correct device or lead failures, adjust programming to improve device longevity and obtain maximum benefit from device-specific pacing or diagnostic features, and recognize battery depletion in a timely manner.

Pacemaker follow-up can be divided into three phases: early postimplantation, maintenance, and end of life.

The main goal of early postimplantation follow-up is to identify and correct any complications of the implantation procedure, such as hemothorax, pneumothorax, cardiac tamponade, lead dislodgement, wound hematomas, and infections. Patients usually stay in a telemetry unit for 24 hours after implantation of a permanent pacemaker. The components of immediate and predischarge follow-up are shown in **Table 11.1**.

While the predischarge PA and lateral chest x-ray are helpful to rule out early lead dislodgement, this complication can also occur several weeks after the implantation procedure. Lead dislodgment usually presents with a sudden increase in the pacing and sensing thresholds, but it can also present as atrial tachycardia or VT triggered by movement of the pacing lead in the atrium or ventricle, respectively (proarrhythmic effect). Rapid identification of lead dislodgement is critical for successful repositioning of the dislodged lead and to avoid proarrhythmia.

Early postdischarge and long-term follow-up usually are performed in specialized pacemaker clinics. Follow-up usually is performed by a specialized pacemaker nurse under the supervision of a physician. In the clinic, device follow-up is performed with the

Table 11.1 Post-Implantation Procedures

Post-implantation Procedures	Comments
Portable chest x-ray	To rule out pneumothorax/hemothorax (mainly observed with the subclavian approach).
PA and lateral chest x-ray	To establish baseline device/lead position and rule out early lead dislodgement.
Pre-discharge interrogation	To verify adequate pacemaker function and selection of pacing mode. Alternatively, an ECG with and without a magnet can be performed to verify adequate pacemaker function before discharge.
Evaluation of pacemaker wound	To exclude early hematoma formation that might warrant modification of anticoagulation or might require a pressure dressing and/or hematoma evacuation.
Patient education	Emphasis should be given to wound care and limitations in physical activity. It is our practice to recommend restriction of shoulder motion to less than 90° and avoidance of heavy lifting in the first few weeks after implantation to minimize the chance of early lead dislodgement.

aid of a manufacturer-specific programmer that allows interrogation of the pacemaker as well as programming of the pacemaker according to the individual patient's pacing needs.

The main goals in the pacemaker clinic are to determine adequate pacemaker function, optimize pacemaker therapy, and identify and treat rhythm abnormalities. Patients may be asked to come to clinic for a wound check or to remove staples, if they were used to close the pocket, 1–2 weeks after implantation. The initial visit to the clinic for device interrogation takes place approximately 6–8 weeks after pacemaker implantation. There may be an initial rise in pacing thresholds in the first 2–4 weeks, after which they tend to decline somewhat. Thus, thresholds checked at 6–8 weeks are more reflective of what the chronic pacing thresholds will be, and pacing outputs can be adjusted accordingly.

In the chronic phase, patients are followed every 6 to 12 months until battery depletion is expected in the near future, which can be determined by the information provided on battery status and projected longevity from the pacemaker interrogation. Close to the end of battery life, patients will require more frequent follow-up, every 1 to 3 months until RRT/ERI is observed during interrogation. Many of these in-office follow-up visits may be replaced by remote follow-up, either transtelephonically or Internet-based (see the end of this chapter for details).

Approach to Follow-Up

The typical pacemaker follow-up visit consists of the following:

1. Question the patient about symptoms that might indicate pacemaker malfunction or the need for reprogramming, complications of the pacemaker implantation procedure, or progression of the patient's overall medical condition. Patients are asked about pain or drainage at the implantation site, which could indicate impending erosion or infection, respectively. Patients are also questioned about symptoms such as syncope or near syncope that might indicate pacemaker malfunction, such as lead dislodgement or fracture.

2. Interrogate the pacemaker after placement of the programmer wand over the pacemaker (**Table 11.2**). For some manufacturers now, the telemetry range of the programmer makes actual placement of the wand over the pacemaker unnecessary. The initial interrogation provides information about the integrity of overall pacemaker function as well as information on cardiac arrhythmias detected during the time interval in between follow-up appointments. In addition, pacing thresholds are determined, sensing is evaluated, impedance is measured, and diagnostics are reviewed. This initial encounter is usually performed by a specialized nurse, nurse practitioner, or

Table 11.2   Information Obtained with the Initial Interrogation

Patient/Pacemaker Information

Battery Status

Last Measured Threshold(s)

P- and R-Wave Measurements

Threshold Trend

Impedance Trend

Parameter Summary

Heart Rate Histograms

Pacing % Counters

Event Counters

physician's assistant. If all components of the pacemaker are working properly and no significant arrhythmia is detected, a final report is printed and saved on a floppy disk.

If any abnormality is noted on the initial evaluation, the physician is notified and the patient is evaluated further before discharge. For example, patients with elevated impedances and high pacing and sensing thresholds may require pacemaker lead revision, since these findings could indicate lead fracture and/or a loose set screw. Similarly, detection of cardiac arrhythmias could require changes in medical therapy and/or reassessment of the patient's condition.

Changes in specific programmed features are usually determined by the supervising physician. For example, patients with excessive ventricular pacing on follow-up could benefit from programming longer AV delays or a lower minimum pacing rate.

Device reprogramming is also beneficial to optimize pacemaker function, prolong device longevity and troubleshoot other problems that do not require revision of the pacemaker pocket or leads.

3. Schedule a follow-up appointment and complete record-keeping. At the end of the visit, the printed report and the disk are filed in the patient's medical record. Doctors often keep a separate folder containing all the information pertinent to the patient's pacemaker. Some institutions also have a computerized filing system where all the device information is kept. These systems are particularly important in the rapid identification of patients affected by manufacturers' advisories (see the following).

Patients with pacemakers functioning adequately are seen every 6–12 months in person, with remote follow-up at 1–3 month intervals in between office visits (see previous information). Patients with cardiac arrhythmias, problems detected by device diagnostics, and/or those affected by device advisories are followed more frequently at the discretion of the clinic's supervising physician.

The goals of pacemaker follow-up are to optimize pacemaker function, recognize complications related to pacing therapy, identify and correct device or lead failures, adjust programming to improve device longevity, diagnose arrhythmias, and recognize battery depletion in a timely manner.

Device Advisories

Pacemaker and implantable defibrillator advisories are issued to notify physicians and patients of potential device malfunction. Pacemaker clinics have an important role in the follow-up of patients affected by a device advisory. Many advisories are issued despite less than 1 percent chance of device malfunction. Device advisories are frequent and can affect a large number of patients. Decisions to explant a normally functioning device because of the potential for malfunction will depend on the likelihood and type of potential failure, individual need for pacing therapy, the patient's comorbidities, and the risk of the explantation procedure. For example, in pacemaker-dependent patients, device failures could have serious deleterious effects and these patients might benefit from early device replacement. On the other hand, patients who are not dependent on their pacemakers can often be followed up closely and intervention postponed until a failure is identified.

> **Pacemaker advisories are issued to notify physicians and patients of potential device malfunction. Decisions to explant a normally functioning device because of the potential for malfunction will depend on the likelihood of failure, patient-specific pacing needs, the patient's comorbidities, and the risk of the explantation procedure.**

Interrogation

Interrogation of most of the data stored in the pacemaker is accomplished either automatically or manually after placement of the programmer wand over the pacemaker. Following a successful interrogation, a report based on this interrogation is printed (initial report). The initial report usually includes the information shown in Table 11.2.

Battery Status and Projected Longevity

The initial interrogation report displays a message describing the battery status as "OK" or "Replace Pacemaker" based on the battery voltage and internal impedance measurements. It also provides an estimate of the time in years or months remaining until pacemaker replacement will be required. This estimate is based on the programmed parameter settings and the percentage of time pacing is required; patients who are paced 100 percent of the time will necessarily have a shorter estimated remaining battery life (**Figure 11.1**).

Lead Impedance

Impedance measurements are taken periodically in each chamber that is being paced. The maximum, minimum, and average lead impedances are recorded every 7 days. Impedance measurements

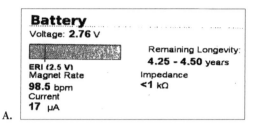

A.

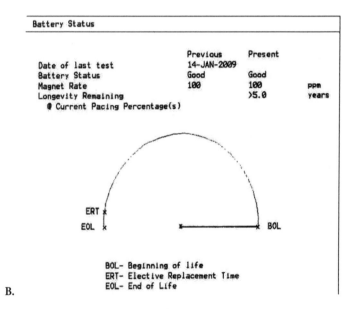

B.

■ **Figure 11.1   Battery status and estimated device longevity**

Device manufacturers have different methods to display this information, as shown by **A** versus **B**.

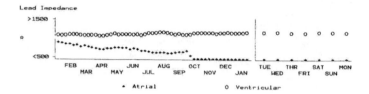

■ **Figure 11.2   Lead impedance trend**

Notice the decrease in the atrial lead impedance below 200 ohms, suggestive of an insulation break.

provide important information about the integrity of the pacing leads. Low impedances (<200 ohms) usually indicate insulation breaks, and high impedances (>1600 ohms) usually indicate lead fractures or loose set screws (**Figure 11.2**).

> **Impedance measurements provide important information about the integrity of the pacing leads.**

Sensing Thresholds

The sensing threshold is the measured amplitude in mV of the atrial (P wave) or the ventricular (R wave) depolarization at the electrode site. This measurement can be performed from the distal to the proximal electrode of the pacing lead (bipolar) or from the distal electrode to the pulse generator (unipolar). The lower the amplitude of the measured P or R waves, the lower the sensing thresholds. In general, acceptable chronic sensing thresholds are P waves greater than 1 mV and R waves greater than 5 mV. Sensing thresholds can be performed manually by the operator or automatically by the pacemaker (**Figure 11.3**). Bipolar sensing is usually preferred. Unipolar sensing may be used in cases of low amplitude P or R waves, if it results in better sensing. However, unipolar sensing is more susceptible to oversensing (such as detection of myopotentials), which can lead to inhibition of pacing.

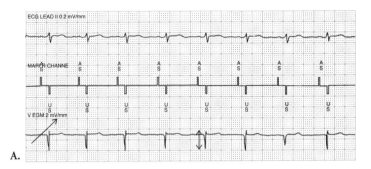

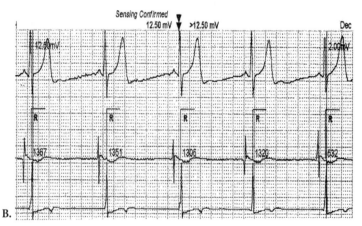

■ **Figure 11.3   Sensing thresholds**

A. Sensing thresholds can be manually determined by measuring the amplitude of the sensed signals if a scale is provided (diagonal arrow). For example, the measured amplitude of the R wave in the ventricular EGM is 10 mm (vertical arrow), therefore, the sensing threshold for the R wave is 20 mV (2mV/mm scale).

B. Sensing thresholds can also be automatically determined by the programmer. The sensitivity setting is automatically adjusted, and loss of sensing indicates the amplitude of the intrinsic signal.

Measurement of sensing thresholds requires spontaneous or intrinsic electrical activity in the atria or the ventricles. This usually requires temporary inhibition of pacing or transient reduction in the lower pacing rate to identify intrinsic activity. Pacemaker-dependent patients may not exhibit any intrinsic activity and may become highly symptomatic with excessively low heart rates or prolonged inhibition of pacing. Thus, determination of sensing thresholds may not be possible in some patients.

Programmed atrial and ventricular sensitivity refers to the minimum amplitude of the P or R wave the device can interpret as spontaneous or intrinsic activity and should not be confused with the sensing thresholds; however, they are closely linked. Thus, a programmed sensitivity of 0.6 mV in the atrial channel means that the pacemaker will not detect spontaneous electrical activity less than 0.6 mV. If the sensed P wave has an amplitude lower than that, it might be intermittently undersensed. Programming the atrial sensitivity to 0.3 mV (increasing device sensitivity) could prevent undersensing, but could increase oversensing of far-field signals and noise.

> Sensing thresholds refer to the measured amplitude in mV of atrial (P wave) and ventricular (R wave) depolarizations at the electrode site. Programmed sensitivity refers to the minimum amplitude of the P or R wave the device will interpret as spontaneous or intrinsic activity.

Pacing Thresholds

The pacing threshold refers to the minimum pacing output that results in atrial or ventricular capture. The pacing output is a function of the voltage amplitude and the duration (pulse width) of the pacing stimulus. Pacing outputs are usually programmed at a 2:1 safety margin. That is, the programmed pacing output is double the pacing threshold to avoid failure to capture during transient and dynamic changes in pacing thresholds. Threshold measurements can be performed from the distal to the proximal electrode in the pacing lead (bipolar) or from the distal electrode to the pulse generator (unipolar). In general, acceptable chronic pacing thresholds are less than 2 volts at a 0.5 msec pulse width (**Figure 11.4**).

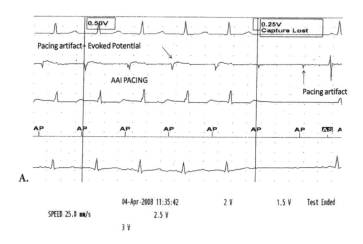

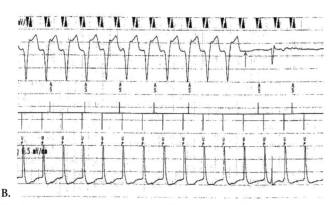

■ **Figure 11.4   Determination of pacing thresholds**

A. The atrium is paced in the AAI mode, with a gradual decrement in pacing output until loss of capture is observed. Consistent capture is observed at 0.5 V at 0.5 msec (pacing artifact followed by an evoked potential; diagonal arrow). When the pacing output is decreased to 0.25 V at 0.5 msec, loss of capture is observed (pacing artifact without evoked potential; vertical arrow). Thus, the atrial pacing threshold is 0.5 V at 0.5 msec (minimal output associated with consistent capture).

B. Pacing the ventricle in the VVI mode, pacing output is decreased gradually until loss of capture is observed (arrow). The ventricular pacing threshold is 2 V at 0.5 msec (minimal output associated with consistent capture).

Pacing thresholds can be performed manually by the operator or automatically by the pacemaker. Elevated pacing thresholds will mandate programming of higher pacing outputs. However, high pacing outputs can significantly shorten the device longevity.

Automatic Capture Management (Autocapture)

Modern pacemakers have algorithms that allow constant adaptation of pacing outputs to a minimal energy to ensure pacing, coupled with continuous monitoring of the pacing thresholds to detect loss of capture and deliver back-up pacing pulses when loss of capture occurs. Clinical studies have proven the safety and efficacy of these algorithms. Constant adaptation of pacing outputs has the potential to increase pulse generator longevity and reduce the cost of pacing therapy significantly. Clinical studies have shown that device longevity can increase more than 50 percent.

Pacing thresholds refer to the minimum pacing output that can result in atrial or ventricular capture. Autocapture algorithms allow constant adaptation of the pacing outputs to a minimal energy to ensure pacing, which can potentially increase device longevity significantly.

Diagnostic Functions

Modern pacemakers can monitor the patient's cardiac rhythm continuously and can record information on cardiac arrhythmias using manufacturer-specific algorithms for the detection and storage of arrhythmias. Accurate diagnosis of asymptomatic and symptomatic cardiac arrhythmias is an essential component of pacemaker follow-up.

Diagnosis of cardiac arrhythmias has important therapeutic implications. For example, patients with asymptomatic paroxysmal AF could benefit from anticoagulation with warfarin, depending on their $CHADS_2$ score for thromboembolic risk. Similarly, patients with runs of nonsustained and sustained ventricular arrhythmias usually require additional cardiac evaluation and might need an upgrade to an ICD, depending on symptoms and LVEF.

The diagnostic features in modern pacemakers also provide an opportunity for correlation between a patient's symptoms and cardiac arrhythmias. Correlation between symptoms and arrhythmias can be sought at the time of interrogation, because arrhythmia episodes are usually logged with the date and time or with patient-activated storage of EGMs by magnet application over the pacemaker at the time of symptoms. Clinical studies have shown that more than one-third of patients may have asymptomatic tachyarrhythmia episodes, and up to two-thirds experience symptoms that do not correlate with a cardiac arrhythmia. Patients with symptomatic or asymptomatic arrhythmias may need arrhythmia-specific treatment, depending on the clinical setting. Those with symptoms but no arrhythmia usually just require reassurance or a noncardiac work-up.

The different diagnostic functions in pacemakers include event counters, histograms, AMS, and stored intracardiac EGMs.

> **Pacemakers can detect and store information on cardiac arrhythmias and allow correlation with a patient's symptoms. Diagnosis of asymptomatic and symptomatic cardiac arrhythmias has important therapeutic implications.**

Event Counters

Event counters provide the number or percentage of paced and sensed events, the number of premature atrial contractions (PACs) and PVCs, and the number of activations of pacemaker-specific algorithms, such as mode switching. The counters thus provide important information about the cumulative percentage of pacing in each cardiac chamber. One can then determine the need to perform programming changes to avoid inhibition of the patient's intrinsic rhythm and minimize cardiac pacing when possible (**Figure 11.5**).

Reduction of cardiac pacing has two goals. The first is to reduce pacemaker-induced ventricular dyssynchrony. This is an achievable

A.

```
Counters
─────────────────────────────────────────────────────────────

Date of Last Reset              14-JAN-2009
                                                 Since Last
                                                 Reset
Paced and Sensed
  A-sensed / V-sensed               11 %           2.2M
  A-sensed / V-paced                43 %           8.4M
  A-paced / V-sensed                10 %           1.9M
  A-paced / V-paced                 36 %           6.9M

Atrial
  Paced                             68 %          13.1M
  Sensed                            32 %           6.3M

Ventricular
  Paced                             79 %          15.4M
  Sensed                            21 %           4.1M

A-Tachy Response
  Mode Switches                                     19
  Total Time                        19 %          1.1 days
  Maximum Time                                    2.8 hours
  Average Time                                    1.4 hours

Ectopic Beats
  PACs                                             4.2K
  Single or Double PVCs                            2.4K
  Three or More PVCs                                3
  Atrial Tachy Detections                          10
  Ventricular Tachy Detections                      2

Ventricular Interval Variation
  Variation        0 <= 10 %                       2.8M
  Variation       11 <= 20 %                     217.7K
  Variation       21 <= 30 %                      62.2K
  Variation          >  30 %                      31.1K

Rate Hysteresis
  Searches                                         3.0K
  Successful Searches                              140
AV Hysteresis
  Searches                                         1.5K
  Successful Searches                               7

Pacemaker Wenckebach Counters                       7
```

■ Figure 11.5   Event counters

Event counters provide the number or percentage of paced and sensed events, as well as the number of PACs and PVCs. (**A**) Event counter information presented in numerical form.

goal in patients with sick sinus syndrome and preserved AV nodal conduction. The second goal is to improve device longevity.

The information provided by the event counters can also help the physician in the assessment of the need for pacing therapy and determination of the severity of the rhythm abnormality requiring

B.

Events

AP Counts   **27%**
VP Counts   **13%**
AV Conduction Counts   **86%**

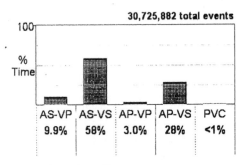

■ **Figure 11.5** (Continued)

(**B**) Event counter information presented as a histogram/graph.

pacing. For example, patients with adequately programmed devices and a cumulative percentage of pacing close to 100 percent are considered pacemaker dependent.

Significant changes in event counters compared to the previous pacemaker follow-up may indicate inappropriate programming, pacemaker malfunction, or a change in the patient's underlying rhythm or condition. One example would be an increase in the number of PVCs, which might be indicative of deterioration in left ventricular systolic function. However, the information provided by the event counters is influenced by a myriad of factors that can affect their accuracy, such as oversensing, undersensing, far-field sensing, interference, cross-talk, and programmed detection criteria. For example, the recorded events might include oversensed events like far-field signals, myopotentials, or EMI. Similarly, undersensing of atrial or ventricular activity could underestimate the incidence of arrhythmias. Due to these limitations, correlation of event counters with stored EGMs is critical for accurate diagnosis and treatment of cardiac arrhythmias.

> Event counters provide the number or percentage of paced and sensed events that could indicate the need for programming changes to reduce pacing. They also provide the number of PACs and PVCs and more sustained arrhythmias that could reflect a change in the patient's rhythm or condition that might require medical intervention.

Histograms

Event histograms provide similar information to event counters, but they are displayed as bar graphs. Heart rate histograms show the heart rate range for both chambers during a specific period of time and the percentage of paced and sensed events. Both atrial and ventricular histograms may also display the recorded number of single PACs/PVCs and PAC/PVC runs. Histograms displaying ventricular response during atrial tachyarrhythmias provide important information about the efficacy of rate control therapy.

High-Rate Episodes

High-rate episodes display the date and time of the maximum rate in both chambers, the average rate in the opposite cardiac chamber, and the duration of the episodes.

Automatic Mode Switching

The ventricular response of dual-chamber pacemakers depends on the atrial rate; thus, rapid ventricular pacing can occur in dual-chamber pacemakers during atrial tachyarrhythmias. The automatic change from a tracking pacing mode (VDD, DDD) to a nontracking pacing mode (DDI, VVI) is called AMS. The main goal of AMS is to avoid rapid ventricular pacing during paroxysmal atrial tachyarrhythmias. AMS algorithms require programs for detection of the initiation and termination of atrial tachyarrhythmias, providing important information about the frequency and duration of atrial tachyarrhythmia episodes. Frequent and prolonged atrial tachyarrhythmias could require changes in medical therapy (antiarrhythmic drugs) or electrophysiologic evaluation (ablation therapy).

AMS is also influenced by oversensing, undersensing, far-field sensing, interference, and programmed detection criteria. For example, a high atrial sensitivity setting can cause sensing of far-field signals or noise that can trigger AMS; low atrial sensitivity can cause undersensing of AF and failure to mode switch, which can lead to rapid ventricular pacing during paroxysmal AF. Due to these limitations, correlation of AMS episodes with stored EGMs is essential for accurate diagnosis of cardiac arrhythmias.

> **AMS avoids rapid ventricular pacing during paroxysmal atrial tachyarrhythmias. AMS algorithms also provide information regarding the frequency and duration of arrhythmia episodes. Frequent and prolonged atrial tachyarrhythmias may require further evaluation and therapy.**

Stored Electrograms

Events counters, histograms, and AMS episodes reflect what the pacemaker has detected, but they can be affected by oversensing, undersensing, and programmed detection criteria. Hence, as already noted, correlation of detected events with stored intracardiac EGMs is essential for correct diagnosis and treatment of cardiac arrhythmias. In one clinical study, stored EGMs confirmed 7 percent of VT episodes, 25 percent of nonsustained VT events, and 35 percent of atrial tachyarrhythmia episodes. The information provided by stored EGMs has important clinical implications. For example, EGMs can confirm the presence or absence of paroxysmal AF and determine the need for anticoagulation therapy. Episodes of sustained or nonsustained VT are not confirmed by EGMs in the majority of cases; thus, without EGMs, patients with "presumed" sustained or nonsustained VT on event counters might require electrophysiologic evaluation to clarify this finding further.

Stored EGMs typically include marker annotations, marker intervals, and the intracardiac EGMs. These three components are usually superimposed to facilitate interpretation of intracardiac signals and increase the accuracy of the diagnosis of cardiac arrhythmias (**Figure 11.6**).

Marker annotations depict pacemaker operation by showing events as classified by the pacemaker and are coded as paced or sensed events in either cardiac chamber. Marker intervals display the interval, in milliseconds, between events. The EGMs can display activity in both cardiac chambers (dual or summed EGMs) or in either chamber alone (Figure 11.6). Stored EGMs also provide the date and time of the event, allowing correlation of EGMs and the patient's symptoms.

Modern pacemakers can store 40 to 120 sec of EGMs once predetermined or nominal collection criteria are met. The number of collected EGMs varies depending on the number of channels recorded and the selected duration of each EGM. Usually, equal portions of preonset and postdetection information are collected. Collection of EGMs can be triggered by high atrial rates/mode switch episodes and high ventricular rates or combinations of both. Events for which EGMs are stored may be triggered by satisfaction of programmed detection criteria or by magnet application by the patient over the pacemaker at the time of symptoms.

Although EGMs can be very valuable in arrhythmia detection and interpretation, programming stored EGMs increases battery current drain and may shorten the time to the RRT (see Chapter 5).

Event counters, histograms, and AMS episodes are affected by oversensing, undersensing, and programmed detection criteria. Hence, correlation of detected events with stored intracardiac EGMs is essential for correct diagnosis and treatment of cardiac arrhythmias.

A.

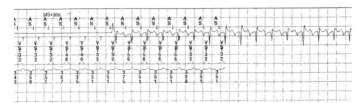

B.

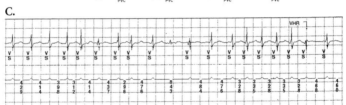

C.

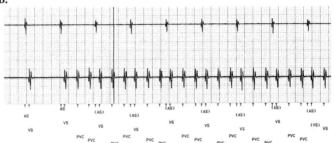

■ **Figure 11.6 Stored electrograms**

Stored EGMs typically include marker annotations, marker intervals, and the intracardiac EGMs.

A. A mode switch (MS) episode is triggered by a 1:1 tachycardia, as demonstrated by the summed EGM (combination of atrial and ventricular signals in a single EGM). AS=atrial sensed event; VS=ventricular sensed event.

B. VT. The atrial EGM is on top and the ventricular EGM on the bottom. There is AV dissociation, with the ventricular rate greater than the atrial rate. The notation (AS) indicates an atrial sensed event that falls in the refractory period.

C. AF. Notice the irregular R-R intervals that trigger detection of a ventricular high-rate (VHR) event.

Device Longevity

The longevity of permanent pacemakers is significantly affected by the programmed pacing rate, stimulation output energy, cumulative percentage of pacing in each cardiac chamber, battery chemistry and capacity, and by the average current drain. Increasing pacemaker longevity could significantly decrease the number of pulse generator replacement procedures and, therefore, decrease cost and procedure-related complications. In addition, optimization of pacing therapy with reduction of unnecessary pacing, as well as the use of autocapture algorithms and pacemakers with high battery capacity can significantly increase device longevity and, hence, improve patient outcomes.

Recommended Replacement Time and End of Service

Determination of the RRT is based on the continuous increase of battery impedance during the discharge process. With increasing cell impedance, the terminal voltage of the battery decreases as a function of current drain. If the voltage falls below certain limit values, prespecified by each manufacturer, the RRT is reached. At this point, the battery voltage has dropped to the point that adequate pulse generator operation will be maintained for a nominal period of 6 months before the output pulse amplitude drops to its EOS value. Exact prediction of EOS is not possible, because measuring battery impedance only provides a rough estimation of remaining service life. Therefore, it is common practice to schedule elective pulse generator replacement once the RRT is reached. Occasionally, patients might present at EOS; immediate pulse generator replacement is usually required in such cases. As mentioned in Chapter 5, the ERI is another commonly used term, and it indicates that approximately 90 days of battery life remain. The term EOL is equivalent to EOS.

Elective pulse generator replacement is recommended once the RRT is reached.

Transtelephonic Pacemaker Monitoring

Transtelephonic pacemaker monitoring (TTM) was introduced in the early 1970s and remains a safe and reliable alternative to in-office pacemaker follow-up. However, TTM is not as effective as in-office or Internet-based monitoring (IBM) systems, given the sophisticated diagnostic capabilities of modern pacemakers. A TTM session typically includes transmission via telephone of an ECG rhythm strip with and without a magnet. The ECG without magnet application shows current pacemaker operation (sensing and/or pacing). Application of the magnet inhibits sensing and thus initiates asynchronous pacing, which will permit analysis of capture if pacing was inhibited by the spontaneous heart rate during the nonmagnet recording. In addition, magnet application allows determination of battery status; that is, every pacemaker model has a specific magnet rate at BOL and a different (lower) magnet rate at RRT or ERI. There are manufacturer- and model-specific transitions from BOL to RRT or ERI (for example, abrupt versus gradual declines in magnet rates as the battery is depleted).

TTM allows for convenient monitoring of pacemaker function and battery status between office visits. Once pacemaker parameters have been optimized, stable patients may be seen in the office once or twice a year, with TTM every 1–3 months between visits.

TTM provides limited but valuable information on pacemaker function between office visits. Data obtained include current free-running pacemaker operation, analysis of capture with magnet application, and determination of battery status.

Internet-Based Monitoring

The expanding indications and growing complexity of pacemakers as well as changing trends in device performance and advisories have significantly impacted device follow-up policies. Currently, the same information that would be obtained during a routine in-office interrogation of an ICD can be transmitted by modem to specialized centers. This information is then sent to the physician/pacemaker clinic via the Internet or fax. However, programming changes still require an in-office visit. IBM allows frequent monitoring of patients affected by device advisories and could facilitate early detection of device malfunction or rhythm changes that could necessitate immediate attention. This service is gradually being expanded to include permanent pacemakers.

> **IBM provides similar information to that obtained during in-office interrogation of implantable devices. The convenience of the system will allow frequent monitoring of patients affected by device advisories and could facilitate earlier detection of device malfunction or rhythm changes that might require immediate attention.**

Suggested Readings

Carlson MD, Wilkoff BL, Maisel WH, et al. Recommendations from the Heart Rhythm Society Task Force on Device Performance Policies and Guidelines Endorsed by the American College of Cardiology Foundation (ACCF) and the American Heart Association (AHA) and the International Coalition of Pacing and Electrophysiology Organizations (COPE). *Heart Rhythm.* 2006;3:1250–1273.

Nowak P. Pacemaker stored electrograms: Teaching us what is really going on in our patients. *Pacing Clin Electrophysiol.* 2002;25:838–849.

Waktare JE, Malik M. Holter, loop recorder, and event counter capabilities of implanted devices. *Pacing Clin Electrophysiol.* 1997;20:2658–2669.

12 ▪ Pacemaker Troubleshooting

GUSTAVO LOPERA, MD, AND ANNE B. CURTIS, MD

Identification and correction of pacemaker malfunction is an essential component of the follow-up of patients with permanent pacemakers. Several tools aid the clinician in this regard, such as changes in a patient's clinical condition, abnormalities seen on ECG, Holter or telemetry, and routine pacemaker interrogation. Early recognition of pacemaker malfunction is crucial in pacemaker-dependent patients, because uncorrected pacemaker malfunction can have serious and potentially lethal consequences in such patients.

Overview of Pacemaker Troubleshooting

Pacemaker malfunction can be due to: (1) component malfunction or failure, (2) inadequate programming, or (3) EMI. Component malfunction or failure refers to any intermittent or constant abnormal function of any of the pacemaker generator's components or the pacing leads. Failure of any component of the pulse generator usually requires the removal and replacement of the generator, but in some instances, the problem might be partially corrected or isolated with pacemaker reprogramming, depending on the type of problem and the patient's individual needs. Inadequate programming and EMI can cause pacemaker malfunction that usually can be corrected by reprogramming and avoidance of the source of EMI. Pacemaker malfunction should be distinguished from ECG findings that look like pacemaker malfunction (pseudo malfunction), but actually represent normal pacemaker function. For example, apparent nonsensing can occur when a retrograde P wave after a PVC resets the pacemaker timing. Pseudo malfunctions result from pulse generator design features. They either do not require intervention or they may be corrected by pacemaker repro-gramming if necessary.

Pacemaker interrogation provides detailed information on pacemaker performance in the time interval between routine pacemaker follow-up sessions. Modern pacemakers automatically determine lead impedances and pacing and sensing thresholds, and they also detect and store information on cardiac arrhythmias (see Chapter 11). Careful evaluation of the information derived from the pacemaker interrogation along with detailed evaluation of a patient's clinical condition and symptoms will aid the clinician in the identification and correction of any pacemaker malfunction. Syncope, near syncope, palpitations, shortness of breath, and fatigue are the most frequently reported symptoms in patients with pacemaker malfunction. However, pacemaker malfunctions can be intermittent and not associated with any symptoms, particularly in nonpacemaker-dependent patients.

Careful evaluation of the patient's clinical condition and information from the pacemaker interrogation are the keys to identifying and correcting pacemaker malfunctions.

Loss of Capture

The surface ECG and the intracardiac EGM signals of a paced heartbeat are the result of the pacemaker polarization artifact and the evoked response. A polarization artifact that is not followed by an evoked response or depolarization demonstrates loss of capture or failure to capture (**Figure 12.1**). Capture in any cardiac chamber is a function of the pulse width and the voltage amplitude of the pacing stimulus.

The most frequent cause of loss of capture is lead dislodgement, which usually occurs in the first days to weeks after implantation. Lead dislodgement may be manifested as a change in lead position on the chest x-ray compared to the baseline postimplantation chest x-ray, an increase in pacing and sensing thresholds, and/or a change in lead impedance. Lead dislodgement can also manifest as a tach-

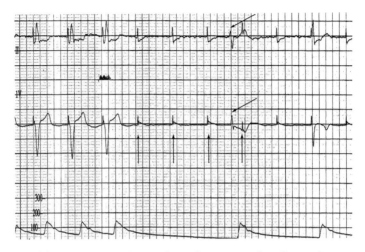

■ **Figure 12.1   Intermittent loss of capture and undersensing**

Vertical arrows show pacing artifacts failing to provoke a ventricular depolarization. Diagonal arrow shows an escape beat that is not sensed by the pacemaker and fails to inhibit the pacing output (undersensing, fourth vertical arrow).

yarrhythmia due to mechanical irritation of the cardiac chamber by a freely moving lead. Lead repositioning will usually be required. Dislodgement of the atrial lead into the right ventricle can, on rare occasions, pace the ventricle and produce unusual ECG patterns; evaluation of marker channels at the time of interrogation can help to identify this problem (**Figure 12.2**).

Microdislodgment of a pacing lead indicates that the lead position on a chest x-ray is unchanged from implantation, yet pacing and/or sensing thresholds have deteriorated, often with a change in pacing impedance as well. This problem may be hard to differentiate clinically from exit block when it first becomes apparent in the weeks following implantation. Exit block is caused by excessive fibrosis at the electrode-myocardial interface and most often is manifested as an increase in pacing threshold with minimal change in pacing impedance. Fortunately, exit block is rare today with steroid-eluting leads.

A.

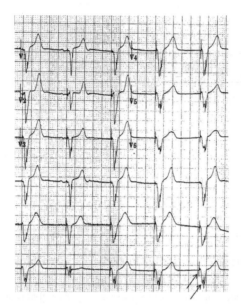

B.

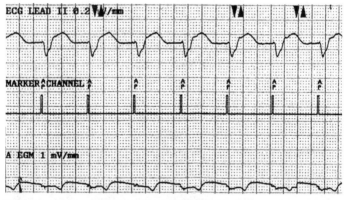

■ **Figure 12.2   Atrial lead dislodgement**

A. Pacing outputs to the atrial lead cause ventricular depolarization. The ventricular lead pacing artifact falls 160 msec after the atrial pacing artifact (double pacing artifact per each QRS, arrows). The fine vertical lines above V1-V6 denote a surface ECG transition and do not represent pacing artifacts.

B. Interrogation confirms ventricular pacing while pacing in the AAI mode (AP = atrial pacing).

Lead fractures and insulation breaks can also cause loss of capture. Typically, lead fracture presents as a marked rise in pacing and sensing thresholds or frank loss of capture. Interrogation of the pacemaker will typically show pacing impedance >2000 ohms and excessive noise on the intracardiac signals during real-time evaluation or during stored EGMs. Insulation breaks can have a similar presentation, but the pacing impedances are usually <200 ohms.

> **Identification of the specific cause of loss of capture requires a detailed evaluation of the clinical information, chest x-ray, ECG, and device interrogation. Particular attention should be given to lead impedance and real-time or stored EGMs.**

Myocardial damage at the electrode-myocardium interface due to myocardial infarction, infiltrative heart disease, or cardiac defibrillation can also cause rises in pacing and sensing thresholds or loss of capture.

Early or late chamber perforation by any type lead can also present with a rise in pacing and sensing thresholds or loss of capture; lead impedance can increase but it usually measures <2000 ohms. Lead perforation may be associated with hemodynamic compromise due to cardiac tamponade or pericardial effusion.

Disconnection of the lead from the pulse generator header (loose set screw) can cause loss of capture or failure of output if completely disconnected. Lead impedances are typically >2000 ohms. Evaluation of intracardiac signals is key in differentiating this problem from lead fracture; noise is usually prominent in lead fracture, but minimal or nonexistent in loose set screw cases. Moreover, lead fracture usually occurs late, whereas a loose set screw presents relatively early postimplantation.

Metabolic abnormalities and drugs, especially hyperkalemia and antiarrhythmic medications, can increase pacing thresholds and, therefore, may cause loss of capture. Antiarrhythmic drugs that can increase pacing thresholds include those from class IA (quinidine, procainamide, disopyramide) and IC (flecainide, propafenone).

Table 12.1 summarizes the most common causes of loss of capture.

Table 12.1   Causes of Loss of Capture

ETIOLOGY	COMMENTS
Lead dislodgement	Change in lead position on the chest x-ray associated with acute rise in pacing and sensing thresholds or loss of capture and no change in lead impedance.
Lead fracture	Rise in pacing and sensing thresholds or loss of capture, pacing impedance >2000 ohms, and excessive noise in real-time or stored EGMs.
Insulation break	Rise in pacing and sensing thresholds or loss of capture; pacing impedance <200 ohms.
Damage to the electrode-myocardium interface	Myocardial infarction, infiltrative heart disease or cardiac defibrillation can damage the electrode-myocardium interface and cause rises in pacing and sensing thresholds or loss of capture. Impedance is usually not affected.
Chamber perforation	Rise in pacing and sensing thresholds or loss of capture; lead impedance can increase but usually <2000 ohms. Cardiac tamponade or pericardial effusion is often observed.
Loose set screw	Can cause loss of capture or failure to output if completely disconnected. Lead impedance is typically >2000 ohms.
Metabolic abnormalities and drugs	Hyperkalemia and Class IA and IC antiarrhythmic drugs can cause an increase in pacing threshold and loss of capture.

Early loss of capture is usually due to lead dislodgement, cardiac perforation, or a loose set screw. Late loss of capture is usually due to lead fracture or insulation breaks.

Sensing Problems

Reliable sensing of intracardiac signals is a requirement for adequate detection of cardiac arrhythmias and for satisfactory pacemaker inhibition or triggering in the presence (inhibition) or absence (triggering) of intrinsic cardiac signals. The components of a sensing system in cardiac devices include amplification, filtering, rectification, and thresholding. Filters typically reject signals with frequencies <10 Hz and >60Hz. After amplification and filtering, the EGM signal is rectified to eliminate the effects of signal polarity and then compared with a sensing threshold. The circuitry recognizes the intracardiac signal when the EGM voltage exceeds the device programmed sensitivity (sensing threshold or minimal voltage required for sensing). As discussed in Chapter 7, the sensing threshold is the measured amplitude in mV of an intracardiac signal or EGM at the electrode site, while the programmed sensitivity is the minimum amplitude of the P or R wave the device can interpret as spontaneous or intrinsic activity.

Cardiac devices also incorporate blanking periods (no sensing) and refractory periods (events are sensed but do not affect pacemaker timing cycles) after each depolarization to prevent sensing of multiple events after a single depolarization. Modern pacemakers also incorporate tachycardia detection algorithms that require short blanking and refractory periods to allow detection of cardiac arrhythmias with shorter cycle lengths. However, these algorithms can also increase the incidence of sensing abnormalities.

Sensing abnormalities are a product of the normal or abnormal interaction of the sensed EGM, the programmed sensitivity (sensing threshold or minimal voltage required for sensing), and the device blanking and refractory periods. Sensing abnormalities can be classified as undersensing or oversensing.

Whether a sensed intracardiac EGM will affect pacemaker behavior depends on the amplitude of the signal compared to the programmed sensitivity setting as well as the timing of the sensed signal compared to any blanking periods or refractory periods.

Undersensing

Undersensing refers to transient or continuous lack of sensing of intrinsic cardiac activity; it results in pacing outputs or stimuli competing with intrinsic cardiac activity (**Figure 12.3**). Theoretically, a concern with pacing stimuli occurring during atrial or ventricular repolarizations is that they may cause AF or ventricular fibrillation in extremely rare occasions. Fortunately, induction of ventricular fibrillation usually requires higher energy outputs than the outputs commonly used for pacing.

Undersensing is the transient or continuous lack of sensing of intrinsic cardiac activity that results in pacing stimuli competing with intrinsic cardiac activity.

Undersensing is usually caused by lead dislodgement, suboptimal lead positioning at implantation, insulation breaks, or changes in intrinsic cardiac signals due to conduction abnormalities or cardiac arrhythmias (**Figure 12.4**). For example, the voltage amplitude of AF EGMs is usually smaller than the sinus rhythm EGM. The small signal amplitude during AF can lead to intermittent or continuous undersensing. The result may be tracking of AF at the URL due to failure to mode switch to a nontracking pacing mode; this is most likely to happen if the programmed atrial sensitivity is >1 mV.

Hyperkalemia, battery depletion, and myocardial infarction close to the pacing electrode can also cause undersensing. Magnet application temporarily disables sensing and has a number of uses, such as assessment of battery status, assessment of capture when the patient's rhythm otherwise overrides the pacemaker, and assurance of delivery of pacing outputs when there is a risk of EMI (see later and Chapter 10).

A.

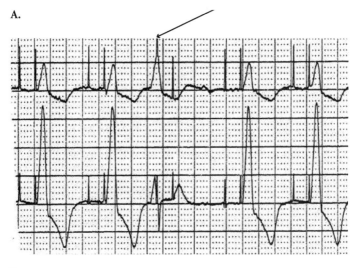

B.

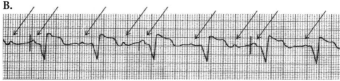

■ Figure 12.3 Undersensing

A. A PVC falling in the blanking period (arrow) fails to inhibit pacing output (functional undersensing or pseudo-malfunction).

B. Intermittent undersensing of P waves. Notice that the first, third, and fifth complexes show P wave undersensing followed by paced P waves (arrows show paced and spontaneous P waves).

Courtesy of Medtronic, Inc.

Modern pacemakers use automatic sensing algorithms to reduce sensing abnormalities. The algorithm periodically monitors the amplitude of the sensed signals and automatically increases or decreases the sensitivity setting to maintain an adequate sensing margin.

Functional undersensing occurs when an intrinsic cardiac event falls in the pacemaker blanking or refractory periods. The

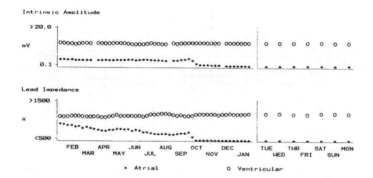

■ **Figure 12.4   Insulation break**

Insulation break causes an increase in atrial sensing threshold (decrease in the sensed amplitude of intrinsic P waves) and an acute drop in atrial lead impedance (< 200 ohms).

result may be abnormal ECG patterns (pseudo malfunction); for example, PVCs falling in the blanking period may fail to inhibit pacing outputs (see Figure 12.3A).

Whatever the cause, most cases of undersensing can be managed with pacemaker reprogramming, by increasing the programmed sensitivity (by decreasing the programmed sensitivity values), by shortening refractory periods in the affected cardiac chamber, or, in some cases, by reprogramming the sensing polarity from bipolar sensing to unipolar sensing. Unipolar sensing can sometimes lead to a greater voltage amplitude of sensed intracardiac signals compared to bipolar sensing. However, unipolar sensing is more susceptible to EMI and myopotentials. It should also be remembered that, while all these maneuvers can decrease undersensing, they can, at the same time, increase the likelihood of oversensing. In a few instances, pulse generator replacement or lead revision may be required to correct undersensing, especially when it is due to lead dislodgement, pulse generator failure, or battery depletion.

Most cases of undersensing can be managed with pacemaker reprogramming by increasing pacemaker sensitivity (by decreasing programmed sensitivity values), by shortening refractory periods in the desired cardiac chamber, or, in some cases, by programming the sensing polarity from bipolar sensing to unipolar sensing.

Oversensing

Oversensing refers to unexpected or inappropriate sensing of intracardiac or extracardiac signals. Oversensing causes inhibition of pacemaker outputs that may result in atrial or ventricular pauses. Such pauses can cause syncope or near syncope, especially in pacemaker-dependent patients. Because inappropriately sensed signals are interpreted by the pacemaker as "intrinsic activity," oversensing can also result in inappropriate mode switching when the sensed physiological or nonphysiological signals occur at a rate that satisfies the tachyarrhythmia detection algorithm (**Figure 12.5**). Some pacemaker models have ATP algorithms that can be triggered by oversensing. Oversensing can result from myopotentials, far-field sensing of signals in a different cardiac chamber, T wave sensing, double or triple counting of QRS signals, or EMI. Oversensing can also result from lead fracture or insulation breaks, but there will usually be associated changes in lead impedances and pacing thresholds, as previously discussed.

Oversensing is the unexpected or inappropriate sensing of intracardiac or extracardiac signals. It can cause inhibition of pacemaker outputs (atrial or ventricular pauses), inappropriate mode switching, and inappropriate triggering of ATP.

Oversensing can be intermittent or constant. Accurate determination of the causes of oversensing requires a detailed evaluation of real-time and stored EGMs and marker channels. If myopotentials

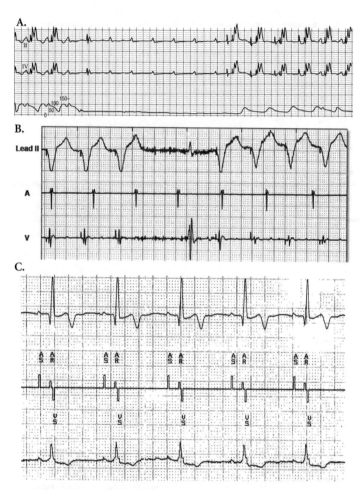

■ Figure 12.5   Oversensing

A. Intermittent oversensing causes transient asystole in a patient with underlying complete heart block.

B. Myopotentials cause oversensing, manifested as short pauses.

C. Far-field oversensing of ventricular signals in the atrial channel is clearly observed in the intracardiac atrial EGM (bottom) and the marker channel (AR) (middle). Top=surface ECG.

(Reproduced with permission from www.cardiosource.com and the American College of Cardiology Foundation) are suspected as a potential cause of oversensing, a series of isometric exercises and pocket manipulation are usually performed to document myopotentials and inappropriate pauses. Pocket manipulation is particularly useful to test the integrity of the leads and the lead connection to the pacemaker header.

Oversensing can be significantly reduced with bipolar sensing and with the use of pacing leads with narrow spacing between the pacing electrodes. Most cases of oversensing can be managed with pacemaker reprogramming by decreasing pacemaker sensitivity (by increasing programmed sensitivity values), lengthening refractory periods in the affected cardiac chamber, and programming the sensing polarity from unipolar sensing to bipolar sensing. In parallel with the previous discussion, programming changes to decrease oversensing can increase undersensing of intrinsic cardiac signals and cardiac arrhythmias. One option available in current pacemakers to try to optimize sensing is automatic PVARP programming. When this feature is activated, the pacemaker determines a value for the PVARP based on the mean atrial rate, shortening the PVARP at high atrial rates to allow adequate tracking of sinus tachycardia and detection of cardiac arrhythmias, and lengthening the PVARP at low atrial rates to protect against PMT.

Pacemakers use automatic sensing algorithms and automatic PVARP programming to reduce sensing abnormalities.

Occasionally, correction of oversensing requires replacement of the pacing lead, mainly in cases of oversensing secondary to lead fracture or insulation breaks. When EMI is the cause of oversensing, avoidance of EMI sources will usually solve the problem.

Table 12.2 summarizes the causes of under- and oversensing.

Most cases of oversensing can be managed with pacemaker reprogramming by decreasing pacemaker sensitivity (by increasing programmed sensitivity values), lengthening refractory periods in the desired cardiac chamber, and programming the sensing polarity from unipolar sensing to bipolar sensing.

Table 12.2   Common Causes of Sensing Abnormalities

TYPE OF SENSING ABNORMALITY	COMMENTS
Undersensing	
Lead dislodgement	Confirmed with chest x-ray
Suboptimal lead positioning at implantation	Manifested as low amplitude P waves or R waves
Small P waves and R waves	Patients with cardiomyopathies or severe chamber dilatation
Insulation break or lead fracture	Associated with changes in lead impedance and pacing threshold
Magnet application	Suspends sensing and triggers asynchronous pacing
Metabolic disorders and drugs	Hyperkalemia and class IC antiarrhythmics can cause undersensing
Battery depletion	Especially severe battery depletion
Damage to electrode-myocardium interface	Myocardial infarction, infiltrative heart disease, or defibrillation can alter the electrode-myocardium interface
Oversensing	
Myopotentials	Can be avoided with bipolar sensing and using leads with narrow interelectrode spacing
Far-field sensing of signals in a different cardiac chamber	Frequently corrected with bipolar sensing, using leads with narrow interelectrode spacing, and avoiding implantation close to the tricuspid annulus and CS
T wave sensing	Generally requires lengthening of the ventricular refractory period, changes in programmed sensitivity values, and/or lead repositioning
Double/triple counting of QRS signals	Usually requires lengthening of the ventricular refractory period and/or changes in programmed sensitivity values
EMI	Corrected by avoidance of EMI sources

Crosstalk

Crosstalk refers to sensing of the pacing stimulus or far-field signals in the opposite cardiac chamber. Typically, it is used to describe sensing of the pacing stimulus or far-field atrial signals in the ventricular channel, which can result in inhibition of the ventricular output and, hence, asystole in pacemaker-dependent patients.

Crosstalk can be reduced or minimized with the incorporation of blanking periods and crosstalk sensing windows during the paced AV interval in dual-chamber systems. Events occurring in the blanking period are not sensed (typically pacing spikes), whereas events sensed in the crosstalk sensing window will trigger a pacing stimulus in the ventricular channel at a shorter and pre-specified AV interval (100–110 msec). The triggered pacing stimulus at a short AV interval will avoid inappropriate inhibition of the ventricular channel and also avoid the potential for a ventricular pacing stimulus to fall on the T wave of a PVC, which could cause a ventricular arrhythmia. This feature is known as ventricular safety pacing.

Electromagnetic Interference

Patients with cardiac devices are subject to numerous sources of electromagnetic radiation that can transiently or permanently interfere with or alter normal device function. Electromagnetic fields are the product of electric fields (volts per meter) and magnetic fields (amperes per meter). The band of the electromagnetic spectrum that can interfere with cardiac devices ranges from 10^9 to 10^{11}. EMI can arise from multiple different sources, including radiofrequency waves, microwaves, ionizing and acoustic radiation, and electric current. These EMI sources are present in many different environments, such as the work place, hospitals, airports, shopping malls, and even at home (**Table 12.3**).

Table 12.3   Sources of Electromagnetic Interference

LOCATION	SOURCE	COMMENTS
Home	Ovens, blenders, electronic equipment, radios, TV, DVD players, cell phones, and portable digital players	Interference is usually avoided by keeping at least a 6 inch distance from the source and the pacemaker.
Work	Arc welding, battery-powered power tools, chain saws, drills, running motors, and alternators	Significance of interference at work places depends on the intensity and proximity of the patient to the source. Testing the work environment by the manufacturer's engineers is sometimes required.
Hospital	Electrocautery, cardioversion, MRI, catheter ablation, lithotripsy, radiotherapy, electroconvulsive therapy	See text for details.
Shopping malls and airports	Electronic surveillance systems	Interactions are usually avoided by walking through security systems and avoiding stopping or leaning against these systems.

Sources of EMI include radiofrequency waves, microwaves, ionizing and acoustic radiation, and electric current. They may be found in the work environment, hospitals, airports, shopping malls, and the home.

Modern cardiac devices now incorporate design characteristics to avoid or minimize EMI, including the use of titanium casing around the pulse generator, diodes and noise protection circuitry and algorithms, and narrow spacing between the pacing electrodes to decrease the antenna effect.

EMI can cause inappropriate inhibition of pacing outputs, because the EMI creates an artifact or noise that the pacemaker interprets as intrinsic activity. The result can be asystole and syncope, depending on the duration and magnitude of exposure to the electromagnetic field. EMI sensed by the atrial lead can result in inappropriate mode switching or inappropriate tracking or triggering of pacing outputs in the ventricle (tachycardic response).

Pacemakers have a noise reversion feature to avoid inappropriate pacemaker inhibition when noise is sensed. The pacemaker operation during noise reversion is asynchronous pacing at the lower programmed rate. EMI can activate noise reversion features or reversion to a backup pacing mode with longer or more intense exposure to an electromagnetic field such as electrocautery or defibrillation. The backup behavior is typically the same as the elective replacement behavior. For example, VVI pacing at 65 bpm is the typical pacing mode for one device manufacturer when a pacemaker reaches the ERI, and the same mode and pacing rate is seen when noise reversion leads to the backup pacing mode.

Some electromagnetic sources, such as radiation therapy or magnetic resonance imaging, can cause transient or permanent damage of the electronic or mechanical components of a pacemaker. Some sources of electromagnetic energy (electrocautery, cardioversion, and defibrillation) can be shunted down the lead, resulting in thermal damage to the lead-tissue interface, which can cause a transient or permanent rise in stimulation thresholds. When performing cardioversion or defibrillation in a patient with a pacemaker, the defibrillation paddles should be placed at least 5 cm away from the generator or in an antero-posterior position. Pacemaker interrogation to check pacing thresholds is also recommended after cardioversion.

Cellular phones, portable media players, and electronic surveillance systems can also cause oversensing and noise reversion. Significant interaction with these devices and cardiac pacemakers is usually avoided when cell phones or media players are kept at least 6 inches away from the pacemaker. Patients should be advised to use cell phones by the contralateral ear and to store it in the belt rather than a shirt or coat pocket over the pacemaker. In regard to surveillance systems, significant interactions with pacemakers are usually avoided by walking through security systems and avoiding stopping or leaning against these systems.

Electrocautery is frequently used in the operating room. Patients with pacemakers undergoing surgical procedures should have their pacemaker set at a rate lower than the intrinsic heart rate (nonpacemaker-dependent patients) or a fixed rate asynchronous mode (VOO or DOO in pacemaker-dependent patients) prior to the scheduled surgical intervention. After surgery, pacemakers should be interrogated and reprogrammed to the original settings. Pacing and sensing thresholds should be rechecked after surgery.

Pacing inhibition, inability to program, loss of telemetry, "runaway pacemaker," and pulse generator failure have been reported with radiation therapy. Significant interactions can be avoided by limiting the radiation exposure to <2 Gy and shielding the pulse generator or keeping it outside the radiation field. If this is not possible, moving the pulse generator to the opposite site may be required. Continuous telemetry during radiotherapy sessions is recommended for pacemaker-dependent patients.

EMI can cause pacemaker inhibition, inappropriate tracking and mode switch activation, activation of noise reversion, and backup pacing modes. More serious complications, such as damage to the pulse generator, runaway pacemaker, and thermal injuries at the electrode-tissue interface can also occur with some electromagnetic fields.

Pacemaker Syndrome

Pacemaker syndrome is a condition that results from AV dyssynchrony or suboptimal AV synchrony, regardless of pacing mode, with disappearance of symptoms upon restoration of AV synchrony. It is most commonly seen with VVI pacing in patients with normal sinus rhythm. The symptoms of pacemaker syndrome vary from mild to severe. The observed symptoms are due to suboptimal timing of atrial and ventricular contractions, the adverse hemodynamic effects of dyssynchronous contractions, and activation of the autonomic nervous system to adapt to abnormal hemodynamics. Symptoms of pacemaker syndrome include dizziness, shortness of breath, palpitations, and fatigue. More serious symptoms, such as hypotension, syncope, and heart failure, can be observed in a small number of patients.

Patients with single-chamber VVI pacemakers and symptoms consistent with pacemaker syndrome may need an upgrade to dual-chamber DDD pacing to restore AV synchrony. Patients with pacemaker syndrome who already have dual-chamber devices may require optimization of their AV intervals by pacemaker reprogramming. AV dyssynchrony can develop with normally functioning DDDR pacemakers when there is inappropriate mode switching. VDDR pacing can lead to pacemaker syndrome when the intrinsic atrial rate falls below the LRL and VVIR pacing ensues. Inadequate programming of rate responsive pacing can also cause symptoms similar to pacemaker syndrome and should be included in the differential diagnosis. Adjusting rate-responsive pacing according to the individual's level of activity can improve the patient symptoms.

> Pacemaker syndrome is a constellation of rather vague symptoms due to AV dyssynchrony or suboptimal AV synchrony, regardless of the pacing mode. Relief of symptoms with restoration of normal AV synchrony confirms the diagnosis.

Pacemaker-Mediated Tachycardia

PMT results from the sensing of a retrograde P wave by the atrial electrode that then triggers ventricular pacing, with development of an ELT as this sequence is repeated for as long as the retrograde P wave is sensed. The most common initiating event for PMT is a

PVC with retrograde conduction to the atrium. However, PMT can also be triggered by PACs, myopotentials, EMI, or intermittent atrial capture. PMT can only occur when the retrograde conduction time (VA time) exceeds the programmed PVARP. For example, if the programmed PVARP is 200 msec, any retrograde conduction from the ventricle that takes longer than 200 msec to reach the atrial electrode can potentially initiate PMT (see also Chapter 9).

PMT can terminate spontaneously if VA block occurs, or it can be terminated by placing a magnet over the pacemaker. Magnet application suspends sensing, and tachycardia will then terminate when the retrograde P wave is no longer sensed. Modern pacemakers have a PMT termination feature that extends the PVARP to 400 msec or withholds ventricular pacing when a device-specific algorithm detects a predetermined number of ventricular-paced and atrial-sensed events.

PVARP can be programmed at the time of implantation or anytime thereafter. Patients with good VA conduction require longer PVARP intervals to avoid PMT. As previously discussed, long refractory periods can interfere with adequate detection of tachycardias. Automatic PVARP programming prevents PMT by extending the PVARP at lower heart rates while allowing detection of tachycardias by shortening the PVARP at faster heart rates.

PMT results from the sensing of a retrograde P wave that then triggers ventricular pacing, with repetition of this pattern for as long as the retrograde P wave is sensed. PMT can terminate spontaneously, by PMT termination algorithms, or by magnet application.

Runaway Pacemaker

Runaway pacemaker is a rare and potentially lethal form of pacemaker malfunction characterized by sudden and unpredictable rapid pacing at exceedingly fast rates, ranging from 100 bpm to 400 bpm. Pacing rates greater than 2,000 bpm have been reported (**Figure 12.6**).

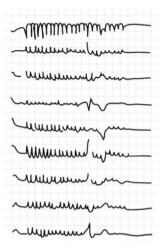

■ **Figure 12.6   Runaway pacemaker causing rapid pacing at exceedingly fast rates**

Adapted with permission from Pugazhendi V, Kedarnath V, Soo GK, et al. Runaway pulse generator malfunction resulting from undetected battery depletion. *PACE*. 2002;25:220–222.

Reported causes of runaway pacemakers include battery depletion, fluid penetration, battery leakage, component failure, stuck accelerometer, electrocautery, and radiation. In order to avoid runaway pacemaker and its attendant consequences, modern pacemakers and ICDs incorporate features such as hermetic sealing, fixed maximum rates, and decreases in pulse amplitude at rapid rates to avoid ventricular capture.

When runaway pacemaker occurs, emergency replacement of the pulse generator is required and could be lifesaving. The problem is solved once the leads are disconnected from the pulse generator.

> **Runaway pacemaker is a rare and potentially lethal form of pacemaker malfunction characterized by sudden and unpredictable rapid pacing at exceedingly fast rates. Emergency replacement of the pulse generator is required.**

Electrocardiogram Interpretation

The 12-lead ECG, telemetry of real-time and stored EGMs, and 24-hour Holter monitors can aid the clinician in the diagnosis of suspected pacemaker malfunctions. ECG interpretation is difficult without knowledge of the programmed mode, URLs and LRLs, and AV intervals. Interpretation is also complicated by the programming of automatic features that can shorten or lengthen the expected pacing intervals, such as sleep function, and shorten or lengthen the AV intervals, such as safety pacing and rate adaptive AV intervals.

Despite all the complex programming features available, pacemakers are rarely programmed to LRL <40 bpm, URL >130 bpm, or AV delays <100 msec. Therefore, exceedingly low or fast heart rates, sinus pauses >1.5 seconds, and inappropriately timed pacing spikes should alert the clinician to possible pacemaker malfunction.

The three basic elements in the ECG interpretation of patients with pacemakers are:

1. Identification of the underlying rhythm
2. Determination of the presence and timing of pacing spikes or the lack thereof, and whether they appear to be appropriate
3. Evaluation of the response to a pacing stimulus (paced, noncaptured, and fusion beats) (**Figure 12.7**)

Identification of the patient's underlying rhythm is important in order to determine the degree to which pacing therapy is needed. For example, patients with spontaneous ventricular rates below the programmed LRL can exhibit excessive cumulative ventricular pacing percentages that have been associated with an increased risk of AF and heart failure. In addition to slow spontaneous ventricular escape rhythms from problems such as an abnormal His-Purkinje system, other causes of high ventricular pacing percentages include a high programmed LRL (>60 bpm) or high doses of negative chronotropic drugs (beta blockers, digoxin, calcium channel blockers). Decreasing the LRL to ≤60

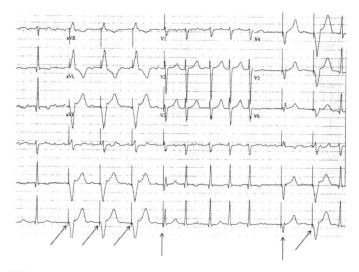

■ **Figure 12.7   Fusion beats**

Vertical arrows show fusion beats; diagonal arrows show ventricular paced beats.

bpm and adjusting the dose of medications with negative chronotropic effects can significantly decrease the cumulative percentage of ventricular pacing and avoid "iatrogenic pacemaker dependency."

Normal pacemaker function requires sensing of intrinsic activity with subsequent inhibition of pacing, with delivery of pacing impulses in the absence of spontaneous electrical activity. Hence, a combination of sensed and paced events is a common occurrence in normally functioning pacemakers (see Figure 12.7). Pacing spikes untimed to intrinsic cardiac events (competitive pacing) usually indicate undersensing, whereas inappropriate inhibition usually indicates oversensing (see Figures 12.3 and 12.5).

The normal response to an appropriately timed pacing stimulus is depolarization of the cardiac chamber where the pacing electrode is located (captured or paced beat). The morphology of the capture beat depends on the location of the pacing electrode within the specific cardiac chamber.

The morphology of a paced P wave depends on the electrode location (narrower in the septum and wider in the lateral wall) and the interatrial delay (the greater the interatrial delay, the wider the P wave). Negative paced P waves in the inferior leads (II, III, and aVF) could indicate lead dislodgement.

The morphology of the paced R wave typically has a LBBB configuration, but pacing in some areas of the right ventricular septum can exhibit a RBBB morphology. Therefore, paced R waves with a RBBB morphology do not necessarily indicate inappropriate placement of a right ventricular lead in the left ventricle; a chest x-ray is required to confirm adequate lead position. Apical positions are associated with wider QRS morphologies than septal positions.

Fusion beats are the result of depolarization of the atria or the ventricles from two fronts, one arising from intrinsic cardiac activity and the other from the pacing electrode. The result is a P or R wave with a "hybrid morphology" as the product of the collision of two depolarizing fronts. Fusion beats do not indicate pacemaker malfunction, since the pacing electrode can only be inhibited after depolarization reaches the electrode site (see Figure 12.7).

> **The three basic elements in the ECG interpretation of patients with pacemakers are: (1) identification of the underlying rhythm; (2) determination of the appropriateness of the lack or presence and timing of pacing spikes; and (3) evaluation of the response to pacing stimuli (paced, noncaptured, and fusion beats).**

Magnet Application

Most pacemakers close a magnetic switch that produces asynchronous pacing (DOO or VOO) at predetermined fixed rates (magnet rates) upon magnet application (magnet mode). The predetermined fixed rate varies depending on the battery voltage and also differs among the different manufacturers. Predetermined magnet rates, according to each manufacturer's specification, are commonly used to determine if the battery is at full capacity (BOL or BOS) or if the battery has reached the predetermined point of battery depletion (RRT, ERI, or EOS).

Asynchronous pacing in response to magnet application is a widely used maneuver to verify atrial and ventricular capture and, hence, to assess pacemaker function. The ability to assess capture and status of the pacemaker battery are the basis for transtelephonic follow-up of pacemakers.

Magnet application at the time of symptoms such as palpitations can also trigger EGM storage and aid the clinician in the assessment of the etiology of symptoms.

Magnet application to pacemakers results in asynchronous pacing at predetermined fixed rates that allows rapid assessment of capture and the status of the pacemaker battery.

Battery Status and End-of-Life Behavior

Routine pacemaker interrogation reports the status of battery voltage and estimated time to replacement. Modern pacemakers provide relatively long battery longevities, up to 12 years or so, even with high percentages of pacing. Obviously, longevity is influenced by pacing thresholds, pacing impedance, and battery drainage secondary to the use of other pacemaker functions.

Premature battery depletion leads to appearance of the ERI indicator <3 years after implantation. With severe battery depletion, the emergence of the ERI indicators will be associated with additional signs of device malfunction, such as failure to output or absence of telemetry.

When the pacemaker reaches a predetermined battery voltage, specific to each manufacturer, an RRT or ERI alert is displayed upon interrogation. At the RRT, the pacemaker generator has about 6 months of life left. From the point that the device reaches ERI, the pacemaker will operate in the VVI mode at a manufacturer-specific rate for approximately 3 months. Diagnostic data collection is suspended at ERI. At the end of 3 months, pacing becomes unpredictable and erratic. The patient should be scheduled for pulse generator replacement shortly after ERI is detected, if it has not already been done in response to an RRT indicator.

At ERI, the pacemaker operates in the VVI mode at predetermined rates for approximately 3 months. Because pacing may become unpredictable and erratic after that time, pulse generator replacement is recommended shortly after ERI is detected.

Suggested Readings

Ellenbogen KA, Gilligan DM, Wood MA, et al. The pacemaker syndrome—a matter of definition. *Am J Cardiol.* 1997;79:1226–1229.

Hayes DL, Vlietstra RE. Pacemaker malfunction. *Ann Intern Med.* 1993;119:828–835.

Sweesy MW. Understanding electromagnetic interference. *Heart Rhythm.* 2004;1:523–524.

13 ▪ Cardiac Resynchronization Therapy

Early reports that AV sequential pacing with a short AV delay could lead to symptomatic improvement in patients with heart failure led to an explosion of interest in pacing therapy for the treatment of heart failure. The initial impression that right ventricular pacing with a short AV delay could be effective in treating heart failure was not confirmed in further investigations. In fact, as is now well known, excessive pacing from the right ventricle has potentially detrimental effects on left ventricular function. On the other hand, CRT with simultaneous or near-simultaneous pacing of both the right and left ventricles has been shown to be effective in the management of patients with heart failure. It is necessary for anyone involved in the care of patients with permanent pacemakers to have some understanding of the indications, programming, and management of patients receiving CRT devices. Implantation of the left ventricular lead is covered in Chapter 6.

Ventricular Dyssynchrony and Mechanisms of CRT

In studies of patients with heart failure, it has been recognized that wide QRS duration correlates with increased mortality. It has been estimated that approximately 30 percent of patients with advanced heart failure have prolonged QRS durations. Usually manifested as LBBB or an intraventricular conduction delay, the resulting late activation of the lateral left ventricular wall compared to the septum and the right ventricle may cause ventricular dyssynchrony. Patients with RBBB do not seem to benefit as much from CRT, because the area with the most delayed activation in this circumstance is the right ventricular outflow tract. There has been some suggestion from small retrospective studies that CRT may be beneficial in some patients with RBBB if there is associated left anterior or posterior fascicular block. However,

there are not enough data at present to make firm recommendations. In borderline cases, echocardiographic evidence of dyssynchrony may be useful to help determine whether CRT may be
beneficial.

Ventricular dyssynchrony has a number of adverse consequences, including paradoxical septal motion, increased duration
of mitral regurgitation, reduced diastolic filling time, and
decreased LVEF, among others (**Table 13.1**). The intention of CRT
is to resynchronize the ventricles with biventricular pacing using a
left ventricular lead in conjunction with a right ventricular lead.
Usually, a right atrial lead is used as well, with AV sequential pacing at an optimized AV delay (see the following), although CRT
has been used in patients with persistent AF as well.

Clinical Trials of CRT

A number of clinical trials have demonstrated the value of CRT in
the treatment of patients with heart failure (**Table 13.2**). The
Multicenter InSync Randomized Clinical Evaluation (MIRACLE)
Trial was one of the pivotal trials in this area. In MIRACLE, patients
with NYHA class III and ambulatory class IV symptoms, sinus
rhythm, QRS ≥130 msec, LVEF ≤35 percent, and left ventricular

Table 13.1	Hemodynamic Consequences of Ventricular Dyssynchrony
Decreased pulse pressure	
Prolonged mitral regurgitation	
Decreased dP/dt	
Decreased cardiac output	
Decreased LVEF	
Reduced diastolic filling time	
Increased left ventricular end systolic and end diastolic volumes	

Table 13.2 Randomized Clinical Trials of Cardiac Resynchronization Therapy

STUDY	DESIGN	NO. OF PATIENTS	MEAN FOLLOW-UP (MONTHS)	RESULTS	P VALUE
MUSTIC (NEJM 2001)	Crossover CRT vs no CRT in patients with CHF NYHA III, EF < 35%, QRS > 150 msec, LVEDD > 60 mm, NSR	58	6	Improved 6MWT QOL Hospitalization Peak V$_{02}$	<0.001 <0.001 <0.05 <0.03
MIRACLE (NEJM 2002)	Parallel arms CRT vs no CRT in patients with CHF NYHA III, EF < 35%, QRS > 130 msec, LVEDD > 55 mm, 6MWT < 450 m, NSR	453	6	Improved 6MWT NYHA class QOL LVEF Peak V$_{02}$	=0.005 <0.001 =0.001 <0.001 =0.009
PATH-CHF (JACC 2002)	Crossover CRT (LV or BiV) vs no CRT in patients with CHF NYHA III-IV, EF < 35%, QRS > 120 msec, PR > 150 msec, NSR	41	12	Improved 6MWT Peak V$_{02}$ QOL NYHA class LV and BiV had similar improvement	=0.03 =0.002 =0.062 <0.001
MIRACLE ICD (JAMA 2003)	Parallel arms ICD/CRT on vs. ICD/CRT off in patients with CHF NYHA III, EF < 35%, QRS > 130 msec, LVEDD > 55 mm, cardiac arrest due to VT/VF, spontaneous VT or inducible VT/VF, NSR	369	6	Improved NYHA class QOL No change 6MWT	=0.007 =0.02 =0.36
CONTAK CD (JACC 2003)	Crossover, parallel controlled CRT vs no CRT in patients undergoing ICD implantation with CHF NYHA II-IV, EF < 35%, QRS > 120 msec, NSR, indications for ICD implantation	490	6	Improved 6MWT Peak V$_{02}$ LVEF LV volumes No significant change NYHA class QOL HF progression	=0.043 =0.030 <0.001 =0.02 =0.10 =0.40 =0.35
PATH-CHF II (JACC 2003)	Crossover CRT (LV only) vs no CRT in patients with CHF NYHA II-IV, EF < 30%, QRS > 120 msec, NSR, Peak V$_{02}$ < 18 ml/min/kg	86	6	Improved 6MWT QOL Peak V$_{02}$ No benefit in QRS 120-150 msec	=0.021 =0.015 <0.001
COMPANION (NEJM 2004)	Parallel arms Optimal Pharmacological Therapy (OPT) vs CRT vs CRT + ICD (CRT-D) in patients with CHF NYHA III-IV, EF ≤35%, QRS > 120 msec	1520	16	Death or hospitalization for CHF reduced by 34% in CRT, 40% in CRT-D As compared to OPT All cause mortality reduced by 36% in CRT-D	<0.002 <0.001 =0.003
			Stopped early by DSMB	24% in CRT	=0.05
CARE-HF (NEJM 2005)	Open label, randomized Medical therapy vs Medical therapy + CRT in patients with CHF NYHA III-IV, EF ≤ 35%, QRS > 120 msec with dyssynchrony (aortic preejection > 140 msec, interventricular mechanical delay > 40 msec, delayed activation of postlateral LV) QRS > 150 msec (no dyssynchrony evidence needed)	814	29.4	All cause mortality/ hospitalization reduction by 37% in CRT All cause mortality reduced by 36% in CRT Improvement in QOL LVEF LVESV NYHA class	<0.001 <0.002 <0.01

6MWT, 6-min walk test; AF, atrial fibrillation; CARE-HF, Cardiac Resynchronization-Heart Failure study group; CHF, congestive heart failure; CONTAK-CD, CONTAK-cardiac defibrillator; COMPANION, Comparison of Medical Therapy, Resynchronization, and Defibrillation Therapies in Heart Failure study group; CRT, cardiac resynchronization therapy; DSMB, data safety monitoring board; EF, ejection fraction; ICD, implantable cardioverter-defibrillator; JACC, Journal of American College of Cardiology; JAMA, Journal of American Medical Association; LVEDD, LV end diastolic diameter; LVESV, LV end systolic volume; MIRACLE, Multicenter Insync Randomized Clinical Evaluation trial; MUSTIC, Multisite Stimulation in Cardiomyopathies study group; NEJM, New England Journal of Medicine; NSR, normal sinus rhythm; NYHA, New York Heart Association; QOL, quality of life; PATH-CHF, Pacing Therapies in Heart Failure study group; VT, ventricular tachycardia; VF, ventricular fibrillation.

Reprinted with permission from Kusumoto FM and Goldschlager NF, eds. *Cardiac Pacing for the Clinician*. New York: Springer, 2008, 2nd edition, pp 432–434.

end diastolic dimension ≥55 mm were randomized to atrial synchronous-biventricular pacing versus no CRT for 6 months. Patients who received biventricular pacing showed improvement in 6-minute hall walk distance, quality of life, and NYHA class.

MUSTIC (Multisite Stimulation in Cardiomyopathy) was a crossover study of patients with NYHA class III symptoms, EF <35 percent, QRS >150 msec, and left ventricular end diastolic dimension >60 mm. This study also showed improvements in 6-minute hall walk distance, quality of life, number of hospitalizations, and peak O_2 consumption. There was also a group of patients studied in MUSTIC who had persistent AF, and similar improvements were seen in those patients.

Other studies of CRT such as PATH-CHF (Pacing Therapies in Congestive Heart Failure), CONTAK CD, MIRACLE ICD (Multicenter InSync ICD Randomized Clinical Evaluation), InSync, and InSync ICD showed functional improvement (exercise capacity, NYHA class, quality of life), left ventricular reverse remodeling (improved LVEF, reduced mitral regurgitation, reduction in left ventricular volumes, etc.), and reduction in hospitalizations for heart failure.

> **Clinical trials of CRT therapy have shown consistent improvements in quality of life, NYHA class, exercise capacity, and ventricular reverse remodeling with biventricular pacing in patients with systolic heart failure and prolonged QRS durations who have NYHA class III–IV symptoms despite optimal medical therapy.**

Mortality and CRT

Two important CRT studies directly addressed the issue of CRT and its effect on mortality. The COMPANION study (Comparison of Medical Therapy, Pacing, and Defibrillation in Heart Failure) randomized patients in a 2:2:1 fashion to CRT-pacing therapy (CRT-P), CRT-defibrillator therapy (CRT-D), or optimal medical therapy (OPT). Eligible patients had to have NYHA class III–IV heart failure, QRS ≥120 msec, and LVEF ≤35 percent. There were 1,520 patients randomized in the study. In addition to improvements in functional status, patients who received either type of CRT device showed a significant reduction in the primary combined endpoint of all-cause mortality and all-cause hospitalization compared to patients treated with medical therapy alone. Patients who received CRT-D therapy had a significant reduction in all-cause mortality compared to the OPT group, with a trend toward lower mortality in the CRT-P patients.

The CARE-HF (Cardiac Resynchronization-Heart Failure) study evaluated the effects of CRT-P therapy alone on morbidity and mortality in heart failure patients. Patients with LVEF ≤35 percent and evidence of dyssynchrony (defined as QRS ≥150 msec or QRS 120–149 msec with echocardiographic evidence of dyssynchrony) were randomized to CRT or optimal medical therapy. The primary endpoint was all-cause mortality or unplanned hospitalization for a major cardiovascular event; CRT was associated with a 37 percent risk reduction (p <0.001). There was also a 36 percent reduction in the secondary endpoint of all-cause mortality (p <0.002) with CRT compared to medical therapy. Thus, CARE-HF was the first clinical trial to demonstrate an improvement in survival with CRT in patients with dyssynchrony and advanced systolic heart failure that was unrelated to any impact from ICDs, which were not used in this study.

CRT reduces mortality in appropriately selected patients with advanced heart failure.

Indications

There is now sufficient evidence of the value of CRT in the management of patients with advanced heart failure that practice guidelines from the major professional societies recommend the use of CRT in properly selected patients. Patients who may benefit from a biventricular device include those with systolic heart failure and an LVEF ≤35 percent, QRS duration ≥120 msec, sinus rhythm, and NYHA class III or ambulatory class IV symptoms despite optimal medical therapy. Such patients are considered to have a class I indication for CRT; in the presence of persistent AF, it is a class IIa indication. QRS duration is used as the marker for dyssynchrony, because this was the criterion specified in the clinical trials of CRT therapy.

Role of Echocardiography in CRT

There are two potential roles for echocardiography in CRT. The first is in the selection of patients for CRT, and the second is in the optimization of therapy after implantation. Optimization will be discussed under follow-up of patients after CRT implantation. With respect to selection of patients for CRT, there is no question that QRS duration is a rather crude measure of dyssynchrony. For this reason, there has been great interest in the use of noninvasive imaging, primarily echocardiography, in the determination of dyssynchrony. A number of parameters have been studied, such as septal-to-posterior wall-motion delay (SPWMD), interventricular dyssynchrony as assessed by the right and left ventricular preejection intervals, and tissue Doppler imaging, in which time to peak velocity in different segments of the ventricle is assessed and a marked delay among them is an indication of dyssynchrony. Abnormal values for various echocardiographic determinants of dyssynchrony are shown in **Table 13.3**.

There have been small studies in which patients with narrow QRS durations (<120 msec) and echocardiographic evidence of dyssynchrony showed significant ventricular reverse remodeling in response to CRT. In addition, while patients with marked QRS prolongation (150 msec) usually have dyssynchrony, patients with moderate QRS prolongation (120–149 msec) may have varying degrees of ventricular dyssynchrony. For this reason, echocardiography is sometimes used to assess the degree of dyssynchrony to

Table 13.3   Some Echocardiographic Parameters of Dyssynchrony

PARAMETER	COMMENT	VALUE
Septal-to-posterior wall motion delay (M-mode)	M-mode; marker of intraventricular dyssynchrony	>130 msec
Tissue Doppler imaging (TDI)	Time to peak velocity in different left ventricle segments	>65 msec
TDI-SD	Standard deviation in time to peak velocity in 12 segments	>32.6 msec
Strain imaging by tissue Doppler imaging	Time consuming image analysis	>130 msec
Delayed aortic ejection time	Marker of interventricular dyssynchrony	>40 msec

determine the likelihood that a patient would benefit from biventricular pacing. The Cardiac Resynchronization Therapy in Patients with Heart Failure and Narrow QRS (RethinQ) Study evaluated the role of echocardiography in the selection of patients for CRT who had QRS durations <130 msec. Patients eligible for the study had NYHA class III heart failure, LVEF <35 percent, and dyssynchrony by echocardiography. Most patients qualified for the study based on tissue Doppler evidence of dyssynchrony. The study was a prospective, randomized, double-blind clinical trial of CRT, with the primary endpoint being the proportion of patients with an increase in peak oxygen consumption of at least 1.0 mg/kg/min with cardiopulmonary exercise testing at 6 months. The results of the study were negative, calling into question the value of CRT in patients with narrow QRS durations despite echocardiographic evidence of dyssynchrony.

At the present time, QRS duration remains the primary criterion for eligibility for CRT in patients with advanced, symptomatic systolic heart failure. Patients with narrow QRS durations (<120 msec), although they may have mechanical dyssynchrony by echocardiography, do not have electrical dyssynchrony and do not appear to benefit from CRT. On the other hand, echocardiographic assessment of dyssynchrony may provide useful adjunctive information in patients with wide QRS durations, especially when the QRS prolongation is due to a nonspecific intraventricular conduction delay or there is borderline widening of the QRS (120–130 msec).

Other imaging modalities such as three-dimensional echocardiography, magnetic resonance imaging, and multiple gated blood pool scintigraphy are under investigation for their utility in the evaluation of patients for CRT, but there is insufficient information at this time to recommend their use.

There is insufficient evidence from clinical studies to support the use of CRT in patients with class III–IV heart failure who have narrow QRS durations, despite echocardiographic evidence of dyssynchrony.

Programming and Follow-Up

Once a patient has a CRT device implanted, it is critical that it be programmed properly for maximum benefit. Since most patients with class III/IV heart failure meet indications for ICD therapy, the CRT devices implanted are most often CRT-D. CRT-P devices without defibrillator capability are used infrequently, either in patients who want the potential symptomatic benefits of CRT but who do not want an ICD (for example, some very elderly patients), or sometimes in patients with moderate left ventricular dysfunction without symptomatic heart failure who require pacing for advanced AV block but who do not meet guidelines for ICD therapy. It should be emphasized that the latter group of patients is not yet indicated for CRT by the most recent practice guidelines, although this is an area under active clinical investigation.

Pacing Thresholds

At the time of lead implantation and at each follow-up visit, the pacing thresholds and impedances of both the right ventricular and the left ventricular leads are determined. While the R wave from the left ventricular lead can be measured, CRT devices use the R wave from the right ventricular lead for sensing. Newer CRT devices allow independent determination of the pacing thresholds from each of the leads. With earlier generation devices, or if for any reason a Y-connector was used to connect the two ventricular leads into a single port in a standard pacemaker, pacing of one ventricular lead alone might not be possible. In such cases, a change in morphology of the paced ventricular beat prior to complete loss of capture can be used to determine that loss of capture on one lead (often the left ventricular lead) has occurred (**Figure 13.1**). If the pacing threshold on the left ventricular lead is so high that reliable capture is not possible, or if diaphragmatic pacing occurs because of proximity of the tip of the pacing lead to the diaphragm or the phrenic nerve, it may be possible to correct the situation by changing the vector for pacing. Many left ventricular leads now have the capability of true bipolar pacing as well as the option to change the vector to unipolar pacing (CRT-P only) or bipolar pacing using the ring of the right ventricular lead. Although some studies have shown that left ventricular pacing alone may be superior to biventricular pacing in some patients, in the overwhelming majority of cases, biventricular pacing is programmed, but with attention to the timing of left ventricular and right ventricular activation (see the following).

With biventricular capture, the ECG in a patient with a CRT device will show a qR or Qr pattern in lead I in 90 percent of patients. Loss of this pattern is highly specific for loss of left ventricular capture. In addition, left ventricular capture alone usually is associated with a tall R wave in lead V1 (**Figure 13.2**).

Pacing thresholds in patients with CRT devices are usually determined individually for each lead. Alternatively, a change in paced morphology with biventricular pacing as output is decreased can be used as an indication of loss of capture in one ventricular lead.

A.

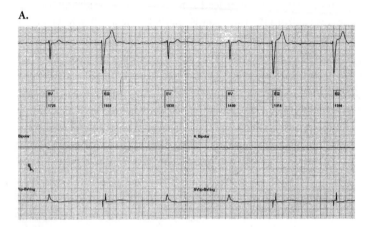

B.

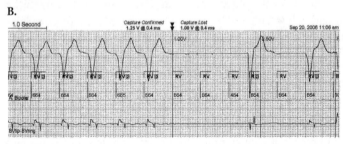

■ **Figure 13.1 Assessment of left ventricular and right ventricular pacing thresholds**

A. Biventricular pacing. From top to bottom: surface ECG lead, atrial EGM, ventricular EGM. R=sensed, R in a black square=sensed in refractory period. The biventricular paced beats (BV) are narrow, while the unpaced beats (RR) are wider with a clear change in morphology.

B. The right ventricular pacing threshold is 1.25 V at 0.4 msec. The intracardiac ventricular EGM on the bottom shows a split signal; the second component is left ventricular activation, which is late with right ventricular-only pacing.

C.

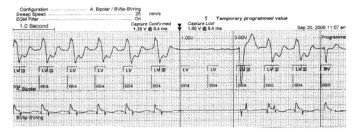

■ Figure 13.1 (Continued)

C. Left ventricular pacing threshold. Note the different morphology on the ECG compared to right ventricular pacing. There is a ventricular escape beat after the two pacing impulses at 1.0V fail to capture the left ventricle.

CRT Programming

In addition to programming pacing outputs based on left ventricular and right ventricular thresholds, the key programming features that need to be considered in a patient with a CRT device are the AV and VV intervals. The AV is generally programmed short, in order to ensure that depolarization of the ventricles is controlled by the two pacing leads, rather than the native conduction system. This is in direct contradistinction to patients with intact AV conduction who have permanent pacemakers, in whom AV intervals are programmed long in order to maximize the use of the native conduction system for ventricular activation.

At the time of device implantation, the AV interval may be programmed to approximately 100–120 msec, which is within a range that provides effective CRT in most patients. Some clinicians perform AV interval optimization in all patients, while others reserve it for patients who do not respond adequately to CRT. AV optimization is accomplished most commonly during echocardiographic examination of the patient. Several different methods have been used for optimization. Pulsed Doppler analysis of transmitral blood flow may be used to determine the optimal relationship between atrial systole and ventricular filling. The goal is to adjust the AV

A.

B.

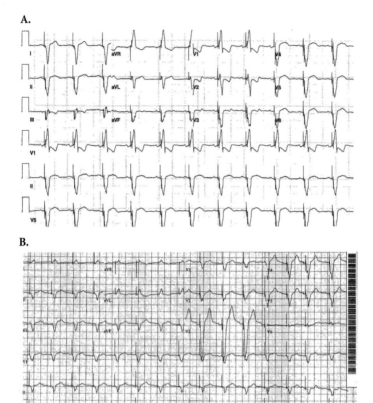

■ Figure 13.2   Electrocardiography of biventricular pacing

A. ECG showing a tall R wave in lead V1 with biventricular pacing. There are two ventricular pacing spikes evident on the ECG. The first one is due to unipolar left ventricular pacing. There is a V-V offset, and the second pacing artifact is from bipolar right ventricular pacing.

B. Right ventricular pacing alone results in a QS pattern in V1.

delay until the A wave (untruncated) occurs at the time of mitral valve closure, which represents the beginning of ventricular contraction. Aside from algorithms developed for use during echocardiography, pacemaker manufacturers have developed algorithms to determine optimal AV intervals based on timing of intracardiac EGMs.

It is also possible to adjust VV timing for CRT. Whereas in most patients, simultaneous pacing or near-simultaneous pacing provides adequate benefit from CRT, in some cases, significant changes in the timing of left ventricular and right ventricular activation are necessary in order for the patient to gain the maximum benefit from resynchronization. Most often, the left ventricle must be activated first to counteract the delay in left ventricular lateral wall activation commonly seen with dyssynchrony. Marked latency in the time from the pacing stimulus to left ventricular depolarization is sometimes seen as the cause of the delayed left ventricular activation. In such cases, preexcitation of the left ventricle is particularly important to achieve adequate resynchronization.

AV and VV optimization should be performed in any patient who fails to respond to CRT, and it is often done in other patients to maximize response to therapy.

Approach to the Nonresponder

Some patients who receive CRT may have almost immediate improvement in symptoms, while other patients take a longer period of time to show a favorable change in NYHA class and functional status. However, one of the challenges of CRT is that a substantial minority of patients, approximately 30 percent, do not have any significant improvement after device implantation. For the patient who does not show a significant response, there are a number of factors to evaluate in addition to issues specifically related to the patient's heart failure and medical treatment. First, the location of the left ventricular lead is critical to achieving resynchronization. The lead should be placed in a lateral or posterolateral branch of the CS. In some patients, technical difficulties prevent placement of the lead where it should be most beneficial. Examples would be small or tortuous posterolateral or posterior branches of the CS. In patients with ischemic cardiomyopathy, scar in the area where the lead should be placed may not allow adequate pacing. In such cases, placing the lead epicardially through a limited thoracotomy or thoracoscopic approach by a surgeon may be preferable to accepting a suboptimal lead position.

For patients who have initial improvement and then experience deterioration in their condition, lead dislodgement is a consideration. A chest x-ray may be helpful in assessing lead position, in addition to determining pacing thresholds on the leads. Lead dislodgement will require reoperation, unless a change in pacing vector or output can correct the problem.

If the lead is in an adequate location, AV and VV optimization should be performed. It is always possible that the patient did not have much dyssynchrony to start with, which may be true particularly if the QRS is only modestly prolonged and assessment for dyssynchrony was not done preoperatively. If significant heart failure symptoms are still present despite optimization, repositioning the left ventricular lead should be considered if the original position was suboptimal. Continued poor functional status despite optimal delivery of CRT may require consideration of approaches other than device-based therapy, such as left ventricular assist devices or even cardiac transplantation.

For the patient who fails to respond to CRT, a number of factors specific to the delivery of therapy should be considered, including suboptimal lead position (including inexcitable scar in the region of the lead), lead dislodgement, and inadequate AV and VV optimization.

Use of CRT in Other Clinical Situations

Atrial Fibrillation

Almost all studies of CRT have required that patients be in sinus rhythm. However, AF is a common problem in patients with heart failure. There have actually been very few studies that addressed the issue of CRT in patients with persistent or permanent AF. Only MUSTIC among the major CRT trials studied a group of patients with AF. MUSTIC included 59 patients with chronic AF, NYHA class III symptoms, a slow ventricular response requiring pacing, and a wide QRS duration. Biventricular VVIR pacemakers were implanted in a randomized, controlled, crossover design study. There were two 3-month treatment periods of VVIR pacing versus biventricular pacing. Only 37 patients completed the study; on-treatment analysis showed improvement in 6-minute hall walk distance, peak oxygen uptake, and a decrease in hospitalization rate.

Clearly, in patients with permanent AF and heart failure who undergo AV junction ablation for the management of a rapid ventricular response, CRT is a better option for long-term pacing than right ventricular pacing. Several studies, involving either upgrading patients with existing pacemakers to CRT devices, or prospective, randomized studies of CRT versus right ventricular pacing, showed that CRT therapy was beneficial in preserving LVEF and improving functional status.

For patients with AF who do not have complete AV block, either iatrogenic or due to native conduction system disease, a key factor governing response to CRT is the degree to which biventricular pacing is achieved. A recent study showed that even achievement of >85 percent biventricular pacing did not lead to functional improvement and ventricular reverse remodeling in patients with AF and intact AV conduction, while patients in sinus rhythm and those in AF who had undergone AV junction ablation showed similar degrees of improvement. The reason for the lack of significant improvement in patients with AF without complete AV block is most likely unrecognized fusion. That is, the irregularity of the ventricular response in AF will allow native conduction to override and suppress biventricular pacing, or compete with it and cause fusion between conduction through the normal conduction system and the two pacing leads. It is important to achieve biventricular pacing >90 percent of the time if the benefits of CRT are to be realized.

> **To provide successful CRT in patients with heart failure and AF, biventricular pacing must be delivered >90 percent of the time. If patients override the pacing because of elevated ventricular rates in AF, and the problem cannot be controlled with medical therapy, AV junction ablation should be considered.**

Class II Patients

While the benefits of CRT have been demonstrated in class III and IV patients, the role of CRT in NYHA class II patients is still under investigation. The preliminary results of the REVERSE Trial have recently been presented. REVERSE was a prospective, randomized, double-blind study of CRT in patients with NYHA class I and II heart failure. The intention was to show whether CRT can prevent or slow progression of heart failure in patients with mild left ventricular dysfunction. Patients were randomized to CRT-on or CRT-off, with the primary endpoint being a composite response indicating progression of disease. The study did not reach statistical significance in the primary endpoint. However, there was some evidence that CRT in such patients may reverse ventricular remodeling and reduce the risk of heart failure hospitalization. CRT in class I–II patients will require further investigation before implementation on a widespread basis can be considered.

> **At the present time, CRT is not indicated in NYHA class I–II heart failure patients.**

Suggested Readings

Abraham WT, Fisher WG, Smith AL, et al. Cardiac resynchronization in chronic heart failure. *N Engl J Med.* 2002;346:1845–1853.

Anderson LJ, Miyazaki C, Sutherland GR, Oh JK. Patient selection and echocardiographic assessment of dyssynchrony in cardiac resynchronization therapy. *Circulation.* 2008;117:2009–2023.

Aranda JM Jr, Woo GW, Schofield RS, et al. Management of heart failure after cardiac resynchronization therapy: Integrating advanced heart failure treatment with optimal device function. *J Am Coll Cardiol.* 2005;46:2193–2198.

Bristow MR, Saxon LA, Boehmer J, et al. Cardiac-resynchronization therapy with or without an implantable defibrillator in advanced chronic heart failure. *N Engl J Med.* 2004;350:2140–2150.

Cleland JG, Daubert JC, Erdmann E, et al. The effect of cardiac resynchronization on morbidity and mortality in heart failure. *N Engl J Med.* 2005;352:1539–1549.

14 ▪ Complications and Lead Extraction

As with any invasive procedure, there are a number of complications that may occur with pacemaker implantation (**Table 14.1**). It is important for anyone involved in pacemaker implantation to be thoroughly familiar with the major complications associated with these procedures, how to minimize the risk of occurrence, and proper management if they occur nonetheless.

Infection

Infection is one of the more serious complications of pacemaker implantation because of its implications for patient management. A pacemaker infection involving the pocket or the leads requires complete removal of all hardware. If a patient presents with signs and symptoms of infection shortly after implantation of a pacemaker, staphylococcus aureus is often the culprit organism. For more indolent infections, staphylococcus epidermidis is frequently the organism that is found on culture. However, other bacteria may also be responsible for pacemaker infections, and so culture of the pocket and leads is necessary in order to make a definitive diagnosis. While removal of recently implanted leads is straightforward, chronically implanted leads are usually much more difficult to remove and require advanced extraction tools. Once the hardware is removed, intravenous antibiotics must be given to eradicate the infection. The duration of therapy may vary anywhere from 2 to 6 weeks, depending on whether it is a localized pocket infection or a systemic infection with positive blood cultures.

The best way to avoid pacemaker infection is scrupulous attention to sterility during the procedure. Prophylactic antibiotics are usually given at the beginning of the procedure, and the pocket is flushed with an antibiotic solution before the generator and leads are placed in it. For a new pacemaker implantation, infection rates

Table 14.1 Complications of Pacemaker Implantation	
COMPLICATION	INCIDENCE
Pneumothorax	1%
Infection	1%
Hematoma	5%
Hematoma requiring reoperation	0.1–0.5%
Subclavian artery puncture	3%
Perforation of the right ventricle	0.1%
Ventricular lead dislodgement	0.5–2.0%
Atrial lead dislodgement	1.5–5.0%
Air embolism	<1%

Table reprinted with permission from Sutton R, Bourgeois I. Techniques of Implantation. In: Sutton R, Bourgeois I, eds. *The Foundations of Cardiac Pacing: An Illustrated Practical Guide to Basic Pacing.* Mount Kisco, NY: Future Publishing, 1991;1(1).

should be <1 percent. If the rate in a laboratory is higher than that, investigation into possible causes should be undertaken. Infection rates with generator changes as well as reoperations for any reason (hematoma, lead dislodgement) are higher than with initial implantations. Since infections associated with generator changes by definition involve chronically implanted leads, this is a common scenario for which a formal lead extraction procedure may be required.

Infection rates for reoperations of any kind (generator change, hematoma evacuation, lead repositioning) are higher than for the initial implantation.

Hematoma

A hematoma may develop because of bleeding from the vascular access site or from the pocket itself. It is important to inspect the pocket carefully before placing the generator and closing the incision site to minimize the risk that the patient will need to be returned to the electrophysiology laboratory for hematoma evacuation. Hematomas are much less common with generator changes, partly because in most cases the existing leads are used and no new vascular access is necessary. In addition, little pocket revision is usually necessary once the pocket is opened and access to the header and leads is achieved.

Most cases of hematomas occur in patients who are on anticoagulation for any reason, typically because of prosthetic heart valves or AF. Mechanical heart valves require that the patient be sufficiently anticoagulated in the perioperative period. There are different approaches that have been used in this regard. Most often, warfarin is stopped several days before the procedure, with unfractionated heparin given as bridging therapy. Heparin is held for 4–6 hours before the procedure, and warfarin and heparin are reinstituted within 12 hours. Of note, current guidelines do not support the use of low molecular weight heparin as bridging therapy in patients with prosthetic heart valves. Alternatively, some physicians now maintain the patient on warfarin through the procedure, perhaps letting the INR drift down to around 2.0 at the time of operation. However, this approach is still somewhat controversial, requiring consideration of factors such as informed consent, the ready availability of recombinant factor VII in the operating suite, and perhaps avoidance of active fixation leads.

Patients who are on warfarin solely for AF and who have no prior history of a thromboembolic event can have their anticoagulation discontinued 3 days before the procedure and then have it reinitiated the day of the procedure. There is no need for bridging with unfractionated or low molecular weight heparin unless there is a history of a thromboembolic event. Patients who are taking aspirin and clopidogrel for coronary stents should be kept on these medications for the time recommended in current guidelines, ideally up to 1 year depending on the type of stent. If the stent was placed more than a year ago, clopidogrel can be stopped 5 days before the procedure and resumed afterward if medically necessary.

Small hematomas are better left alone. If ongoing bleeding is suspected, or a large hematoma causes the patient significant discomfort or causes tension to the incision site, the hematoma should be evacuated. Needle aspiration is generally not advised, because the blood has usually coagulated to the point where aspiration is not possible, and introduction of a needle into the pocket increases the risk of infection.

The need for anticoagulation for other medical conditions is responsible for many hematomas after pacemaker implantation.

Pneumothorax

Pneumothorax is one of the known complications of pacemaker implantation, occurring in approximately 1 percent of cases. It is clearly a risk with the subclavian approach to lead implantation. It is less common with the axillary approach, assuming scrupulous attention is paid to keeping the tip of the needle over the first rib at all times. Pneumothorax is nearly unheard of with a cephalic vein cutdown, which is one of the advantages to this approach.

Pneumothorax may be recognized during the procedure by a change in the patient's oxygen saturation or by a complaint of chest pain or shortness of breath. Fluoroscopy may show that the lung markings do not extend all the way to the chest wall, particularly in the apical region. If a significant pneumothorax develops during the procedure, implantation of the pacemaker may need to be postponed until the pneumothorax is treated. More commonly, the problem is detected on the postoperative portable chest x-ray, or the PA and lateral chest x-ray obtained the day after implantation. If it is small (<10 percent), the patient may simply stay in the hospital an additional day or so for observation. A larger pneumothorax will require the placement of a chest tube, prolonging the hospital stay by several days.

**Pneumothorax is most common with the subclavian approach
to lead implantation, less likely with axillary access, and
extremely rare with a cephalic vein cutdown.**

Lead Dislodgement

Lead dislodgement occurs in <5 percent of pacemaker procedures. The risk of lead dislodgement is one of the reasons for monitoring the patient overnight after the implantation. Lead position is checked with a chest x-ray the morning after the procedure, and the device is usually interrogated as well to determine pacing and sensing thresholds as well as lead impedances. It is possible to have a lead dislodge whether the fixation mechanism is active or passive. Regardless, lead dislodgement requires reoperation and should be performed promptly after it is recognized. A dislodged lead may cause arrhythmias, and it becomes harder to reposition a lead that has been in place for several months.

Cardiac Perforation

Perforation of the heart may occur with placement of a pacing lead. Whenever a patient has a severe drop in blood pressure during a pacemaker implantation procedure, cardiac perforation should be suspected. Fluoroscopy should be performed, which may show enlargement of the cardiac silhouette and lack of movement of the heart border. If tamponade is suspected, an echocardiogram should be ordered stat. A large effusion with hemodynamic compromise requires immediate pericardiocentesis. In the case of right ventricular perforation, there is rarely a need for surgical intervention, because the perforation usually seals over spontaneously. Pericardiocentesis with placement of a drain for several days will usually be sufficient. On the other hand, perforation of the right atrium often requires thoracotomy for closure of the perforation site.

Other Complications

It is possible to cause vascular tear, particularly of the SVC just before it enters the right atrium. In order to minimize the risk of this problem, it is important to be careful as one advances the lead out of the peel-away sheath, so that it makes the turn in the SVC to enter the atrium. Hemopneumothorax may occur with vascular tears, and arterio-venous fistulas may occur as well. Many of these complications will require surgical correction, in some cases emergently.

A problem that can occur most commonly with peel-away sheaths that do not have a diaphragm is air embolism. Just as the guide wire and dilator are removed, and before the lead is advanced in the sheath, air may enter the sheath. If it is recognized promptly (air may be visualized in the vascular system under fluoroscopy), the patient should be placed in the Trendelenberg position and given 100 percent oxygen with a rebreather mask. Usually the patient will exhibit hemodynamic compromise within a couple of minutes of the event, but these measures will help to mitigate the problem.

Malposition of a pacing lead in the left atrium or the left ventricle is possible, either through a patent foramen ovale or with an actual perforation of the septum. It may be difficult on an AP view of the chest to recognize that the lead is malpositioned, because the evaluation of pacing and sensing may be perfectly normal. This problem can be avoided by viewing the lead in the RAO and LAO projections before fixing the lead in place. The possibility of lead malpositioning is also one of the reasons for obtaining a PA and lateral chest x-ray the day after implantation, in order to be sure that the leads take their proper course anteriorly. A recognized malposition of a pacing lead on the left side must be corrected immediately. The lead may be pulled back toward the right side with little risk, and then repositioned in the proper location.

Injury to the tricuspid valve is possible as the lead is advanced through it, although development of significant tricuspid regurgitation as a result of the placement of pacing leads across the valve is fortunately uncommon. Venous thrombosis is another complication from pacemaker implantation, particularly when there are multiple leads in the vein. It is usually manifested as upper extremity edema and is treated with anticoagulation.

Vascular tears, air embolism, inadvertent placement of a lead in the left heart, and injury to the tricuspid valve are all complications that may occur during pacemaker implantation.

Lead Extraction

Lead extraction is performed by many fewer physicians than the number who perform new pacemaker implantations, partly because of the much less frequent need for lead extraction procedures and also because of the skill required to perform the procedure. However, having an understanding of indications for lead extraction and the general approach to the procedure is helpful for those working in electrophysiology laboratories where the procedure is performed.

Indications for Lead Extraction

Infection remains the single most important and absolute indication for lead extraction. When a pacing system becomes infected, whether in the pocket or within the vascular system, the only way to clear the infection completely is to remove the pacemaker generator and leads. It is still not uncommon to see physicians remove the generator from an infected pocket and cut the leads at the entry site into the vascular system. It is difficult to clear the infection completely when hardware is left behind, and cutting the leads in the pocket prevents the use of many of the extraction tools that require a length of exposed lead over which to advance various sheaths and cutting devices.

Another important indication for lead extraction is lack of vascular access for a new lead. This problem usually occurs in a patient who already has one or more leads in a central vein and needs an additional lead placed, either because of malfunction of one of the existing leads or the need for a new lead, such as a left ventricular lead for biventricular pacing. If the vein on the ipsilateral side is occluded, extraction of the malfunctioning lead can be performed, with the sheath that was used for extraction providing the access for a new lead. This approach may be preferable to placing the new lead on the opposite side and tunneling the lead over to the side where the existing leads and generator are. It should be noted that lead extraction is not the only alternative for placement of a new lead when vascular access is difficult. For example, venoplasty can be used when a guide wire can be placed in the vein but stenosis prevents placement of a sheath or lead.

Most other indications for lead extraction are somewhat discretionary, and it is important to weigh the risks and benefits of lead extraction carefully when making a decision. For example, rather than extract a single malfunctioning lead, it may be capped off and left in place, and a new lead implanted. Factors to consider in making such a decision include the age of the patient, the age of the lead, and the number of existing leads. For a very young patient with a life-long need for pacing therapy, it may be preferable to extract any extraneous/malfunctioning lead(s) rather than simply add another lead. One reason is that it is easier to extract a lead that has been in place for a few years than one that has been in place for more than a decade. In addition, such patients may be anticipated to require additional leads throughout life, and so abandoning leads in the vascular system may not be in the patient's best interest. On the other hand, elderly patients with a single nonfunctioning lead are usually best served by abandoning the lead and adding a new one.

Pacemaker leads that have been implanted for less than a year are usually fairly easy to extract, and lead removal should be considered if the lead is no longer functional for any reason and replacement is necessary. Leads that have been in place for many years usually have enough scar tissue built up on them that removal becomes more difficult. In addition, old leads are more likely to break down during the process of extraction, increasing the chances that the lead tip or other material may be left behind.

Finally, the number of leads should be considered. Although there is no absolute number of leads in the vascular system that should not be exceeded, the greater the number of leads, the more likely it will be that vascular occlusion will occur. In addition, interference of one lead with another may be a problem. Although this is less likely to be an issue with pacing leads, defibrillator leads may pick up noise from adjacent abandoned leads that may be interpreted as tachyarrhythmias and lead to inappropriate shocks.

Commonly accepted indications for lead extraction include infection and the need for access for new leads; other indications are considered more discretionary.

General Approach to Lead Extraction

The general approach to lead extraction will be explained here. It is important to understand that lead extraction should only be performed by highly trained individuals. In addition, only a general overview of the technique of lead extraction is provided here to allow medical professionals and trainees working in electrophysiology laboratories an understanding of the procedure and the ability to assist as necessary.

Lead extraction is performed under sterile conditions in an electrophysiology laboratory or in an operating room. The presence of an anesthesiologist may be advisable, even if the patient is simply monitored under conscious sedation, in case rapid response is necessary for hemodynamic collapse. Having a cardiac surgeon on standby is prudent as well.

After local anesthesia is provided to the skin and subcutaneous tissues of the pocket, an incision is made and the generator and leads are dissected free of the pocket. Any sutures around the suture sleeves are cut and removed. It is important to remove all foreign material, and that includes nonabsorbable sutures. If the lead is an active fixation lead, an attempt is made to retract the screw before proceeding further. The end of the lead is cut off with heavy scissors, and the distal insulation is removed with a scalpel. In the case of a coaxial bipolar lead, the outer coil is pulled slightly and cut off, exposing the inner coil and insulation. The insulation on the inner coil is then cut off, allowing access to the inner coil.

One of the principles of lead extraction is that one wants to apply traction to the lead in a controlled manner. After placing a stylet into the lead, one can gently pull on a lead that has been in place for a short period of time, and it often will become free and easily removed. However, if any resistance is met, one should replace the straight stylet with a locking stylet. A locking stylet has a coil or beveled end that can be fixed in the tip of the lead. Then, when one pulls on the stylet, the force is transmitted to the tip of the lead and puts less stress on the proximal lead and insulation. Once the locking stylet is in place, a suture is placed around the lead proximally to keep the insulation and lead bound together.

If traction alone is insufficient to remove the lead, there are various tools that are used to gain access to the vascular system and remove the scar tissue that has built up on the lead and that prevents removal. There are steel (only used for access to the subclavian vein itself), Teflon, and polypropylene sheaths that can be used for mechanical removal of the lead. More commonly, there are laser and electrocautery sheaths that are used for lead extraction (**Figure 14.1**). With a laser sheath, there is an optical fiber within that delivers laser energy around the circumference of the tip of the sheath. The electrocautery sheath has two electrodes at the tip of the sheath close to each other, so that radiofrequency energy is delivered from one point along the sheath, not the entire circumference. In either case, the sheath is advanced over the lead and laser/electrocautery delivered at binding points. When the sheath is advanced close to, but not over, the lead tip, the sheath is

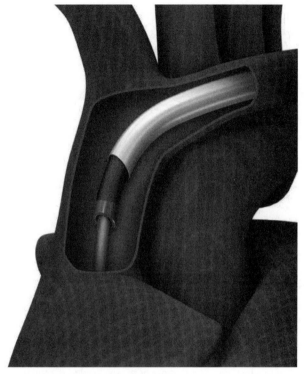

■ Figure 14.1   Laser lead removal

The inner laser sheath is shown being advanced over the lead to be removed. The outer sheath is advanced as adhesions are broken up by the laser.

Reprinted with permission from Spectranetics, Inc.

held steady and countertraction is applied by pulling on the locking stylet. In most cases, the lead will break free of the myocardium and may be removed from the body (**Figure 14.2**). If a new lead is required, the sheath may be used to introduce a guide wire over which a new peel-away sheath may be advanced after removal of the extraction sheath.

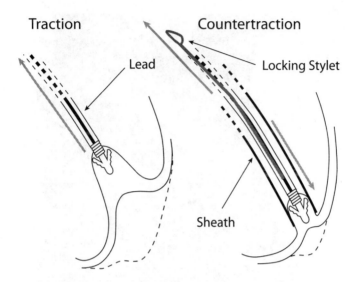

■ Figure 14.2   Countertraction technique

Direct traction on a lead, as shown on the left, puts stress on the myocardium and may increase the chance that rupture will occur. It should only be used for leads that have been in place a short time. Once a sheath has been advanced almost to the tip of the lead, whether it is a mechanical sheath or a laser sheath, that sheath is kept steady as traction is applied to a locking stylet that has been advanced to the tip of the lead (right). The applied countertraction allows removal of the lead with much less risk of myocardial tear.

Reprinted with permission from Spectranetics, Inc.

In some cases, removal of the lead from the superior approach is not possible, often because the lead has previously been cut off in the pocket. In that event, it is possible to remove the lead from the femoral approach. A large sheath is advanced to the atrium from the femoral vein, through which a snare is advanced. The snare is used to grab the body of the lead, and the lead folds on itself as it is pulled into the sheath. The sheath is then advanced to the tip of the lead, and countertraction is used to pull the lead free from the myocardium.

The major risks of lead extraction are vascular tear or cardiac rupture. Even in skilled hands, the possibility of a tear in the subclavian vein with exsanguination into the thorax or cardiac rupture with tamponade is real. In addition, when such complications occur, there is usually a very short period of time in which to intervene to save the patient. In some hospitals, lead extractions are routinely performed in an operating room with a surgeon on standby so that the chest may be opened quickly in the event of an emergency.

After placement of a locking stylet, mechanical, laser, or electrocautery sheaths may be used to break up adhesions on leads to allow countertraction and removal from the vascular system.

Suggested Readings

Byrd CL. Managing device-related complications and transvenous lead extraction. In: Ellenbogen KA, Kay GN, Lau C-P, Wilkoff BL, eds. *Clinical Cardiac Pacing, Defibrillation, and Resynchronization Therapy,* 3rd ed. Philadelphia: Saunders Elsevier; 2007:855-930.

Love CJ, Wilkoff BL, Byrd CL, et al. Recommendations for extraction of chronically implanted transvenous pacing and defibrillator leads: Indications, facilities, training. North American Society of Pacing and Electrophysiology Lead Extraction Conference Faculty. *Pace Clin Electrophysiol.* 2000;23:544–551.

Parsonnet V, Bernstein AD, Lindsay B. Pacemaker implantation complication rates: An analysis of some contributing factors. *J Am Coll Cardiol.* 1989;13:917–921.

Index

A

A2 catheters, multipurpose, 82
AAI pacemaker mode, 99, 101
AAIR pacemaker mode, 99
Ablation therapy, 165
ACC/AHA/HRS 2008 Guidelines for Device-Based Therapy of Cardiac Rhythm Abnormalities, Class I, II, and III indications, 23–24
Acceleration, programming, 115*t*, 117, 119
Accelerometer, 110–112, 111*t*
Acquired AV block
    causes of, 30
    indications for pacing in, 31*t*
Action potential, ECG correlates of, 16
Active fixation, passive fixation vs., 44–48
Active fixation leads
    with fixed screw, *45*
    in right atrium, 49–50
Activities of daily living, programming, 115*t*, 119
Activity sensor
    piezoelectric crystal with, 110–111
    for rate-responsive pacing, 111*t*
Acute myocardial infarction, AV block in, 34*t*
Adams, Robert, 1
Advisories, device, 153–154, 171
AF. *See* Atrial fibrillation
AF "burden," defined, 125, 144
Age of patient, lead extraction decisions related to, 222
Air embolism, pacemaker implantation and, 216*t*, 220
Algorithms
    ATP, 181
    autocapture, 160
    automatic mode switching, 165
    automatic sensing, 179

    for minimizing ventricular pacing, 128
    for modern pacemakers, 158
    pacemaker-mediated tachycardia termination, 128–131
    proprietary, for termination of PMT, 130–131
    rate cut-off, 124
    running average, 124
    for suppression and termination of atrial tachyarrhythmias, 132
    tachycardia detection, 177
American Heart Association, Science Advisory Panel of, 132
Amplification, 179
Amplitude, pacemaker impulse and, 93
AMS. *See* Automatic mode switching
Anesthesia, pacemaker implantation and, 67
Angiographic catheter technique (or outer/inner catheter technique), 84–85
Angiographic technique, for coronary sinus lead placement, *86*
Annotated event markers, 146
Anterior fascicles, left bundle branch, 32
Antiarrhythmic drugs
    atrial tachyarrhythmias and, 165
    loss of capture and, 175–176
Antibiotics, pacemaker infection and, 215
Anticoagulation, hematomas and, 217
AOO mode, 63
Arrhythmias
    AMS response and characteristics of, 125–126
    conduction system disorders and, 21
    lead dislodgement and, 219
Arterio-venous fistulas, 220
Aspirin, 217